Fred's Guide to Stem Cell Transplants

Patient to patient talk and walk
down this cancer path not chosen

Life is good!

Fred & Kathy

Fred & Kathy Roth

outskirts
press

TO:

My Huntsman mentor, Bruce;

My transplant brother, Colton, my fellow patient;

My adopted mother, Tina, Colton's mother;

My Huntsman Cancer Institute transplant amigos, Brian, John, Rand;

The Huntsman Cancer Institute staff: every one of them;

And especially my donor, Chris!

To my new

"Comrade in Cancer Challenge,"

whoever you are.

We now walk this path together.

We are on the same team.

Game on

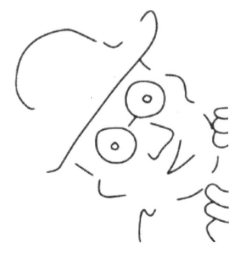

Thanks to our illustrator, Allai Kaushik, a young artist from the Greater San Francisco Bay area. His style ranges from expressive simple line drawings that we requested to detailed pen and ink presentations. He participated in this project with good heart and dedicates this work to his grandfather.

Table of Contents

Hi, I'm Fred

If you have this book, you likely have cancer. This challenge feels big, feels insurmountable, and scares you mightily.

I have been there. And now I'm not! I am here to share my story of a stem-cell transplant, offer suggestions, and cheer you on.

I have embraced the challenges and now pay it forward by mentoring others who find they must walk a path not chosen. I have witnessed and learned much about courage, persistence, and the real strength of others. I want you to benefit from this accumulation of experiences. Someday I hope to hear what worked for you.

This looks like it's all about me. The intention is that it really is all about you.

- In each chapter I share my story.
- I highlight the ideas or actions that worked for me.
- I share some of my personal stats so that you have a point of reference against a patient case.
- I share my thoughts as I worked through each episode and give you space to make your plan.

I advise reading this book in small sections as you progress. Work your way through this book as you work your way through your treatment. Read one section ahead to help you prepare for the next phase of activity. Check the table of contents to help you find information that you might need. Keep it handy. Pick it up when you're curious about the next stage. I hope there's something that will give you a thoughtful perspective to make good decisions.

If you're reading, your show is already on the road. Let's get started.

I encourage you to keep an insurance file and two companion notebooks: a medical journal and an internal journal. Although keeping written records might seem difficult when you are feeling overwhelmed, it gives you pause to process what's happening. It gives you a sense of control. It might save stress from confusion and conflict in the future.

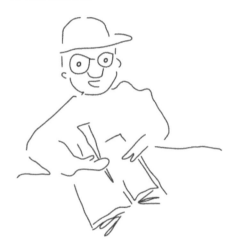

I suggest a file for insurance communications. I kept every statement and every e-mail exchanged with health insurance, disability insurance, and Social Security. Having names, dates, and discussions (verbal notes or printed e-mails) was helpful more than once. Insurance is complicated. People interpret information differently. There are delays between events and billings to confuse any disputed matters further. If you haven't started a file for insurance communications, **start now**.

Your medical journal is your account of your medical experience. I found it very important to have my own records of my conditions, medications, reactions, and other references. It proved to be a valuable reference as the days, weeks, and months started to blur.

Your Medical Journal: Keep track of your daily medical experiences.

- Blood counts:
  - » White blood cells (WBC)
  - » Red blood cell (RBC)
  - » Hemoglobin (HBC)

- » Platelets
- » Absolute Neutrophil Count (ANC)
- New Conditions/Changed conditions
- Medications: added/dropped/dose change
- How you feel
- Observations
- Questions
- Staff of the day
- When in the hospital: keep track of calories and fluids as you approach hospital release
- Milestone appointments—one hundred days, six months, one year, etc.

Your Internal Journal: Process the experience in any quiet, active way you want, but do something tangible.

This time is a wild time for which few experiences have prepared you. Your experiences need to be processed thoughtfully. Thoughts, beliefs, and ideas will swirl fiercely in your mind and through your spirit. Be present. Step back and observe. Be conscious of the words that want to come out for the day. Give your thoughts and feelings the right to be expressed.

Writing is one way you can stop the whirling of your thinking. Your brain might be on "reloop," fixating on the same ideas over and over. To write, you must choose the thought and the words and send them through your fingers to capture them amid many that exist at the same time. I suggest writing by hand, rather than typing. Writing by hand is a physical act and a direct connection between your head and your hand. There's no distraction of spell-check, no temptation to edit as you go. This journal is not an exercise in crafting. Often called expressive writing, this method is just nonstop writing, so that the ideas flow unfiltered. If no ideas present themselves, write "I don't know what to write" until something surfaces. It's your mental work space. It's private. Let whatever happens, happen.

Be a pen and pencil aficionado. Sketch, if it better suits your expression. Many people process with visual images rather than words. It's your private space. Do whatever works as your way of coming to terms with your life's left turn. It's a process of getting your thoughts down on paper so you can look at them—what's true and what's not.

There's enough ahead that carrying rough thoughts is an added burden. Get 'em out; get 'em down, so you can assess the quality of your thinking. You want to be as clear-thinking as you can. Writing helps you climb out of the confusion and become a calmer observer. What's happening? What needs to happen?

This is your day. Don't waste your time on mindlessness. Seize the day, because now time has a different, powerful meaning.

Here are two big questions that need to be addressed up front: What gives meaning to your life? Why bother taking on this fight?

"He who has a WHY to live for can bear almost any HOW."
- Friedrich Nietzsche

Coming To Terms With The Diagnosis

We cannot change the cards we are dealt,
just how we play the hand.
- Randy Pausch

Nothing in life is to be feared, it is only to be understood.
Now is the time to understand more, so that we may fear less.
- Marie Curie

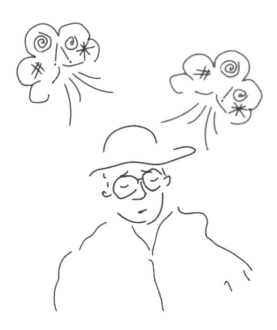

The Diagnosis—Why Me?

We had just celebrated our fortieth wedding anniversary. I'd enjoyed a terrific July 4th that included mountain hiking and lots of activity. On Monday, I hiked early morning and went to the eye doctor. Tuesday, I hiked early morning to Catherine Pass (10,000 ft.), a popular hike in Alta, Utah.

Wednesday I went for my annual physical with a new general physician, a young doctor, since my long-standing GP had retired.

On Friday the 13th, I received a call from the young GP informing me of the blood test results with the three dreaded words, "You have cancer." Further tests were ordered immediately. He sent me to the local hospital where he had connections and indicated that they were expecting me. The diagnosis was acute myeloid leukemia (AML-M6), with the recommendation that I start chemotherapy that day.

AML–M6 is a rare form of leukemia. There is not much information on it, because AML-M6 occurs so infrequently. The doctor explained it with a dance metaphor: "In the ballet of blood, the mother cell emits cells that continue to split and differentiate to the varying forms of red blood cells, white blood cells, and platelets. Somewhere in the process, missteps occur, creating malformed, inefficient cells. Although the cancer is rare, the treatment is the same: remove the inefficient system with chemo and replace the mother cells (stem cells) with the healthy cells of a donor and hope that they happily move into the bone marrow and produce perfection. "

How does one get AML? No one knows. Chemical exposure, radiation exposure, and/or just bad luck. I had some huge positives on my side. I was in good physical condition, at a good weight, and I had no symptoms. The only way the cancer was found was through a routine blood test during my annual physical.

I negotiated a few days before starting chemo in order for my wife to return home from business travel and for me to come to terms with the news. I was off and running on a path not chosen.

Home alone, I wrestled with the night when it occurred to me at 3:00 a.m. that I should check our insurance affiliations. It turned out that the initial hospital, across town, was out-of-network. The Huntsman Cancer Institute (HCI) was nearby and in-network. It was more convenient and had an excellent reputation, and we had friends who had been successfully treated there. In the morning I called the first hospital to indicate my decision to use HCI.

My wife, Kathy, and I notified family and key friends. As a couple we ran through a gauntlet of wild emotions until we realized the only choice was to move forward. We worked on two plans. Plan A: I survived; Plan B: I did not.

We started Plan A: We worked our way through this storm as best we could. We weren't sure what that meant, but we would meet it head on.

We started Plan B: We scrambled to establish household stability. We quickly worked on a household record system and cleaned up "messes" to give us peace of mind.

Before I left for the hospital, I cleaned out a closet and painted it and backed up files on my computer. Why? These mundane tasks gave me a focus as I dealt with the mental chaos of "life threatened."

Nevertheless, this roller coaster was VERY emotional, frightening, and life-changing for Kathy and me. We strived to create a game plan and move forward. We would give it all we had.

Fred's Lessons Learned

For a few days we were in shock with no detailed information. We searched the Internet and quickly learned to be cautious of Internet information. It added confusion and angst, because we did not know what we were viewing or if the information actually applied to me. Many negative statistics were disheartening.

Diagnosis–Shock/Disbelief–Why Me?

- Being negative will not help me get through this. Positivity heals!
- What do we have to do to survive this situation? We went to work developing a positive game plan.
- We had the "what are the dismal odds of survival" discussion with our doctor, and then we moved on. We did not focus on the negative survival prospects. Someone had to be on the positive side of the statistics. It might as well be me.
- We were optimistic and hopeful in spite of all the negatives going on around us. We concluded it was OK to be afraid. We knew this illness was very serious, but we tried to be focused and hopeful.

Reminder to family and friends: the importance of the annual physical. Without my annual physical, I would have detected this cancer much later, and it would have presented a more complicated diagnosis.

Getting your life in order

- Plan A: you survive.
- Plan B: you do not.
- Create peace of mind by having a Plan B ready just in case. My peace of mind was a mad dash to organize before I moved on to my new inpatient world. We had division of household labor. Some things I did; other things Kathy did. We both realized that there were household details that I took care of that would be problematic if I were not here. We scurried to create "the notebook." (We share the organization of this notebook in the appendix.)
- Patient and spouse need to work together to help each other. This situation was traumatic for both of us.
- Have someone accompany you to doctor appointments as an

extra set of ears. Stress adds a layer of confusion between your ears and your brain. You nod. You speak. However, you are not sure what language they are speaking, although you are well aware of the bottom line. Your companion can also help you take notes during the discussions with the doctors and nurses.

- We also realized the importance of having legal documents in order.
  1. Power of Attorney: Lets an appointed person sign for you, if need be, to facilitate family/personal business matters.
  2. Health Care Proxy: Appoints a health-care agent to make decisions for you, should you become incapacitated.
  3. Advanced Directive: Also referred to as a living will, it provides instructions for end-of-life care. Hospitals often want their own forms, for clarity. A hospital social worker can often assist in this matter.
- Thank goodness we had good health insurance. The hospital will help you navigate health-care services. There are many resources to assist. Make sure you understand how health-care expenses will be addressed.
- Get your life in order and then focus on survival.

Fred's Game Plan

I'm in it to win. I will give this fight everything I have, because it is the fight of my life. Whatever the health-care providers ask of me, I will give it to them as best I can. Spending energy stressing about the negatives is wasted energy.

I can't travel this road alone. I appreciate my partner is in this journey. I commit to trying to be respectful of my spouse since I anticipate that I will not always be at my best and may not acknowledge her sincere commitment to my survival. I told Kathy up front, "I apologize now if I become difficult. I am afraid."

I also appreciated that my employer was immediately concerned and supportive. My employer restructured my work responsibilities so I was not distracted.

Your Game Plan—it needs to be your ACTION PLAN.

- Clear the deck of distractions.
- What needs to be addressed to give you peace of mind while you are in your fight?
- List worrisome tasks or issues so others can address them with you and for you.
- Write down those tasks. Delegate the ones you can. Let them go so you can focus on your game plan.
- Have your own method of stabilizing your thinking. Much of your success comes from within. Do something to access your thinking and ideas.

Your Internal Journal

I've got absolutely nothing to lose and everything to gain.

If I had one book to accompany me through the emotions of cancer, it would be *From This Moment On, a Guide for Those Recently Diagnosed with Cancer* by Arlene Cotter (Random House, 1999). This book is a patient-to-patient introduction to your cancer diagnosis that will help prepare you for the challenging days ahead. It is an easy-to-read format of one concept per page with accompanying art. It addresses the internal thought processes in a powerful way. These ideas lend themselves for reflection in your internal journal.

Caregivers, Our Thinking Partners

When someone is walking beside us,
we have more courage to walk into the unknown
and to risk the dark and messy places in our journey.
- Henry Kimsey-House

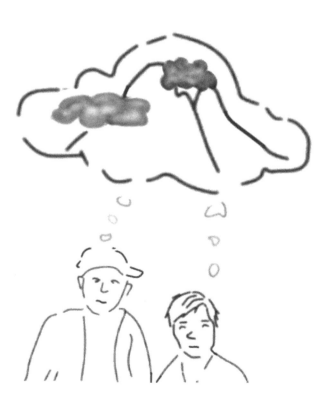

Our Copilots, Our Caregivers-In Appreciation of Caregivers

Our caregivers are our special people who accompany us on this journey. They are our extra ears and a thinking brain when we are overwhelmed. Our copilots need to understand the evolving medical game plan and our personal strategy. They are our cheerleaders when times are tough. They hold us accountable to our personal vision when we want to hibernate. They also attend to home matters. The caregiver role is a stressful, energy-draining, critical role that deserves acknowledgment, appreciation, and consideration.

Core advice for healthy caregivers

The prevalent advice to caregivers is self-care. The human brain loves predictability. The familiar is energy efficient. Habits are life activities on autopilot. There is nothing predictable, familiar, or habitual about being a caregiver during a medical crisis. There are many layers of stress that accumulate over the course of the day. There are the stresses of the patient and absorbing the information of the hospital, staff, insurance, and your patient's changing condition. There is your own stress of traffic, parking, and navigating within a hospital to find food, drink, and restrooms. There is the stress of keeping your household going, paying bills, attending to family members and pets, maybe working a job, and taking care of nagging tasks that accumulate in your normal life. Caregiver burnout can erode your effectiveness in doing any of these things well.

Build a game plan for your own stress relief and support as you see how your caregiver role unfolds. Be conscious of your own good care decisions. It's tempting to default to whatever is easiest. Work out an agreement that allows for caregiver time, place, and space. We found that mornings were busy with medical routines. Our agreement was for Kathy as caregiver to use the mornings at home as she wanted or needed. She exercised, read for pleasure, worked on the computer, did errands, spent time with friends, and maintained the household. It was a time for her to do normal, routine life activities. She admits that sometimes she just "stared at the wall" and didn't do anything. She generally arrived around 1:00 p.m. and spent most of the day thereafter with me at the hospital.

Kathy generally packed her own food so that she controlled her diet. The hot potato bar, wings, onion rings, fries, and other comfort food items were mixed among healthy choices and called loudly when her stress ratcheted up. She found it was better to bring her own cooler with her own food and munched along at dinnertime. Getting run down, adding extra pounds, or needing a haircut only adds to the caregiver's distress.

Caregiver self-graded report card:

- Did I exercise?
- Did I eat fruits and vegetables?
- Did I feel sunshine or breathe fresh air?
- Did I sleep soundly? Do I need a nap?
- Did I laugh and experience joy and gratitude?
- Do I feel supported? Am I supporting others through this community?
- What's my energy level 1 (listless) to 10 (brimming)?
- What's my mood level 1 (low) to 10 (exuberant)?
- What worries me today at the hospital? At home?
- What needs attention?
- Who can help?

Guarding against caregiver burnout

Caregiver burnout has a negative impact on physical, emotional, and spiritual aspects of your well-being. Do any of these symptoms feel familiar?

- A feeling that something bad is going to happen
- Anger
- Anxiety

- Difficulty concentrating
- Difficulty making decisions or problem solving
- Fatigue
- Headaches
- Feelings of tension
- Sleep problems
- Shaking or trembling
- Feelings of sadness or grief

The following website is a strong resource that will address the above symptoms with good information delivered in a quick and easy format: www.helpforcancercaregivers.org

Hospitals understand the stress and strain on caregiving and generally provide support services. Social workers were available for one-on-one discussions or to work through problems that fester at home. We connected with a staff clergy member and benefited from his daily visits. Caseworkers and insurance specialists provided guidance where it was needed. Onsite support groups were available. Community members offered creative activities for eligible patients and caregivers. An art studio provided an additional means of expression. Kathy was sorry she didn't take advantage of the weekly knitting session. It looked like a nice group. It would have been a new skill for her with meditative qualities. This medical world understands the stress of caregiving and is ready and willing to help.

Be The Match, operated by the National Marrow Donor Program (NMDP), offers the Peer Connect program to help with questions and concerns. It will put patients in touch with trained volunteers, who are transplant recipients and caregivers, to answer questions and share tips from their own transplant experience. Peer volunteers are available to talk by phone or e-mail. To request a connection, visit BeTheMatch.org/patient-peerconnect.

Strategies for caregivers as thinking partners

All of us are smarter than one of us. Watch and listen to other caregivers. Many are experienced. They can share strategies that they've learned along the way. We learned lessons by watching others.

Have a plan. How are we going to get through this medical challenge? We worked hard initially to have a shared philosophy and shared language to discuss things. Friends mentioned the Chardi Kala philosophy in conversation that gave us this focus. We share it later in this book. Create a patient game plan that the caregiver can hold up as a model. Have a caregiver plan for commitment of time and energy. This is the time for strong teamwork.

The caregiver needs time and space. The patient needs time and space as well. Everybody likely needs a daily break.

HCI allows families to stay in the patient rooms with family restrooms, shower facilities, and a kitchen in common areas. Few people are accustomed to being together 24/7 without a break. When moms are left with toddlers, they often complain that the only break is when they're in the bathroom. Do we do this to our patients by being ever-present in their rooms?

When you are a constant companion, might you take charge and tap the patient's inner child? If so, you make patients a little less involved and a little less responsible for their own care. They don't get to decide if they commit to walking, meditating, journaling, reading, or drawing. These activities are solitary things that help them come to terms with their situation. Does constant caregiver attention interfere with a patient's inner dialogue? Patients are ultimately responsible for their contribution to treatment and recovery. It is their journey.

Independent time allows for more conversation besides your own. Who talks when the staff is present? Does the patient actively engage with the doctors, or does the caregiver jump into the conversation and become the information provider? Do caregivers inadvertently take over the show in their own need to make it better or fix it?

Patients can feel irritable, frustrated, and angry. These feelings can inadvertently be directed at the caregiver. We all intellectually know the reaction comes from stress, but it can still feel personal. Observe it as a symptom of the circumstance rather than absorb it as a truth about you. Those moments are a good time to consider a break. A break sends a message about boundaries and provides time and space to process the emotions in a more constructive way.

The quiet doubts that linger with the caregiver include the following: If I leave, maybe something will happen. If I'm gone and something does happen, did I fail to provide strength and comfort? If I am here, I'm still part of a couple, a parent.

Patients are concerned about the effects on spouse and family. They may allow constant contact as a way of taking care of the caregiver. It might be difficult for them to initiate the space for fear of appearing ungrateful or rejecting. "How are we going to do this?" starts the conversation about the plan.

Caregivers can save the day. Per the Apple® campaign– "Think Different."

Caregivers need to be objective observers. What's happening? How is my patient handling this? Being supportive does not mean sharing the experience. It often means supporting an alternative thought process. Sometimes the caregiver can disrupt the patient's swift sinking into fear by offering a different message.

One day at a time. The one-day-at-a-time concept makes a big difference. It expands on the interpretation of "Be in the moment. Let go of the past. Don't worry about tomorrow." When conditions might seem to be slipping, it's easy to feel a rising panic and sink into a vortex of fear. Focus on today's facts. Your body works to navigate the world when you are awake. Your body does repair work when you are asleep. Your body will likely bring changed conditions to the next day. Doctors, too, change overnight. Perhaps they had an experience that shifts the way they view your information. Enough evolves that tomorrow brings changing dynamics. The caregiver focuses on a hopeful possibility of tomorrow.

Every body is unique. Every body is a mystery. Others' stories are not your story. Connecting to patients and families naturally leads to caring bonds. All patients and their families have their own stories. Don't internalize their experience as your awaited path. You will be motivated by others who approach this journey with a different energy and strategy. You will be grateful as you hear circumstances more complicated than your own. You will be helped by others. You will help others. There's good energy both ways. But you will walk your own path.

Cancer is not gender specific. Caregivers are both male and female. During our stays we had several young female patients with attentive young husbands. We made an effort to connect with these fellows. They were less likely to connect with other caregivers casually. We often found that they would connect with me as I walked in the halls. They would come to talk when I was available for company. Their instinct was always to present a strong front, regardless of the circumstances. They, too, needed TLC.

Patient and caregiver working together: Stress and the importance of mindset.

We found several discussions about the brain and stress. We thought it was significantly insightful.

There are two general methods of processing stress. People either react to stress or respond to stress.

People **who react** to stress process it at a lower level of the brain, the amygdala/limbic system, considered our ancient brain. It generates fear and is survival based. It works on the basis of fight or flight, freeze or appease. It is a threat mindset.

People **who respond** to stress recognize the fear impulse and take a tiny moment to pause and assess. In that pause they take in the stressful circumstance and consider the next move. The pause to consider operates at a different region of the brain, the prefrontal cortex, where functions such as language and analysis occur. It's a challenge mindset. Every stress event provides the choice to manage it as a threat or challenge. This stress event is a big one!

Kathy noted that I took the challenge mindset. I was not going to solve the science side of my problem. I could take on the health side of my problem. I would do everything I could to maintain health and strength.

Your Internal Journal

Every stress event provides the choice to manage it as a threat or challenge.

How do you think you are addressing the stress of the diagnosis and treatment?

Are you reacting or responding?

Begin The Challenge:
Chemotherapy/Induction

You never know how STRONG you are
until being STRONG is the only choice you have.
- Bob Marley

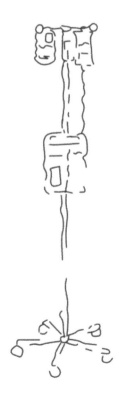

Checking in to the Hospital—Chemo Round 1/Induction

I packed my hospital bag. What do you pack for potentially several weeks in the hospital?

This trip was the first of many clinic visits and hospital stays. The clinic routine: blood draw, temperature, weight, blood pressure, oxygen utilization, then get tucked in a small examining room waiting for test results delivered by a professional.

Good professional practice dictates that doctors stay with you in an appointment as long as it takes for you to understand what's happening. Be patient when your appointment is overdue. Doctors may be attending to patients who are in crisis. You would want their careful attention if you were in crisis.

This is the first time I met the doctor in charge of my case and heard the details of my case as best they knew. The doctor entered the room with the greeting, "So, you are the Olympic athlete that I have heard so much about."

At age sixty-two, I was "old" by leukemia-treatment standards. The mid-level team who conducted my initial interviews and tests were enthusiastic about my chances. I was in good health, at a good weight, and with good vital statistics. I walked in under my own power. Many people my age arrive by ambulance because they passed out from lack of oxygen from limited red blood cells. He recommended aggressive treatment. If I were in poor health or poor condition, though, they would have only made me comfortable for my remaining months.

To his credit, our doctor stayed with us until we did not have any more questions. He did not act rushed to leave to see his next patient until we were satisfied with the next step.

I moved into my new room and met a variety of professionals who all came in with paperwork, information, and notebooks to begin the process. By 6:00 p.m., I had a chemo pole and bags of chemicals connected to my arm with tubing. It's weird, but it's manageable. I was scheduled for seven days of chemotherapy. This first round is referred to as induction chemotherapy.

My new daily hospital routine: Blood draws occurred around 4:00 a.m. There was the routine of taking my temperature, blood pressure, and oxygen levels every four hours. There was a bustle of activity, so I decided I might as well get up, get washed and dressed, and go for a walk in the hall, dragging my pole alongside me. I could order breakfast at any time off a menu. I ate each morning around 7:00 a.m.

The team of doctors arrived when the blood tests results were available. I was on my feet ready with questions. I recorded in my medical journal all the daily data, including how I felt and any issues and medications. I started a separate spreadsheet of blood-count test results. I kept this practice beyond the hospital stay and continue it for ongoing clinic visits to this day.

Every day I had an assigned nurse, health care assistants (HCAs), and a cleaning team, as well as a team of doctors. Everyone was equally important. The HCAs collected data. The nurse administered and watched for change. The doctors interpreted tests, blood readings, and observations. Cleanliness is absolutely critical when your immune system is shut down. The food service staff was at my beck and call. All these people were part of my lifeline and support team. I needed them all. I did what I could to help them do their jobs well. I intended to be a respectful, appreciative and cheerful patient even when I was struggling.

I wanted to be a respected member of the team. I supplied information that no one else had: how I felt. I was attuned to the importance of being accurate about what I was feeling. I understood that there was no value in being stoic and macho with regard to pain. Pain was a symptom that needed to be reported. It would have been easy to say I was feeling well when I was actually hurting or tired.

My goal was never to have the doctors see me in bed. I was dressed in my own clean clothes (sweat pants, T-shirt, and sweat shirt) and standing when doctors arrived. I would have my report and my questions ready for them each day. I never wanted the doctors to see me in bed, and they DID NOT for the entire ninety-three days (over the course of seven months) I was in the hospital. In those instances when the medication made me drowsy (i.e. Benadryl during blood transfusions), I would doze in the recliner until the effect wore off.

Once my overall game plan started coming together, I started to think about goals beyond my hospital room. I established short-term goals that were about experiencing the daily riches of life. I started to hone long-term goals. Given the gift of more time, how do I want to use this time? All of this planning added fuel to my motivation fire.

Fred's Lessons Learned

- This was a tough game to "go it alone." The fear factor was high. The conversations and vocabulary were foreign. I thought I knew what was happening but I was not confident that I was taking in all the information and understanding it as I agreed to the next steps.
- I did not know what questions to ask. "What does that mean?" and "I don't understand" were good questions to start with. When you think you've got it, repeat it back in your own words. Be engaged.
- Kathy helped me process the medical information and added another opinion to decisions. Nurses were also my champions. They observed my condition, understood the terminology, and helped clarify the communication between the doctors and me.
- I tried to be an active participant in "rounds" during the daily medical staff visits. I prepared my own assessment based on how I was feeling. I had questions prepared. This little routine made me feel I was a person versus medical specimen and that I was part of the team.
- I was honest with the doctors about how I felt so they could provide accurate treatment based on my current condition. I wasn't macho and didn't hide my problems. I could have been withholding valuable information.

- As rounds concluded, I asked the doctors for their summary statement on my status. This feedback was good. It confirmed what I was doing well or indicated the day's focus. I jotted it down in my medical journal and went to work doing what was needed.
  Examples:
  - » We're watching this problem. (aware and accessing)
  - » You're responding as expected. (reassuring!)
  - » You need to drink more liquids. (instructive)
  - » Fantastic progress—keep it up! (encouraging!)

Your Internal Journal

Mind, Body, Spirit

A young resident doctor said to us, "We are trying our hardest to understand the body. We bring our collective body of knowledge. The mind! The spirit! These are powers we don't know how to harness. We don't know how to turn these into prescriptions, treatments, or therapies, but we know they play powerful roles."

You, the patient, are at the controls of these extraordinary powers. Explore your powers. Use your journal to explore your thinking. Listen to your inner self. Fear is fearsome! The use of language by talking or writing lifts your thinking out of the fear mindset and into a higher form of processing.

- What kind of patient are you preparing to be?
- How do you see your part in this health journey?
- Start honing your goals for the day, for your inpatient stay, and for life beyond the hospital.

The First Week of Chemo

I wondered how I would react to chemo. I remembered the movie *Bucket List*. Jack Nicholson relished a great dinner and then spent all night with his head in the toilet. Events such as this one will happen at some point, and you will end up laughing about it later with your new cancer friends.

I fumbled with the chemo pole, my constant companion and "dancing partner." Kathy quickly decided to call the pole Ginger. Get it? Fred and Ginger? Younger staff members had no concept of Fred and Ginger. Several staff members said they remembered their grandparents talking about Fred and Ginger. It provided many quirky YouTube moments where we introduced these young people to this iconic dance team.

I got into the rhythm of my new community. When I was not communicating with my team, I was out in the hallway walking. It was part of my "good health/stay strong" objective.

I made my bed early, even though the HCAs changed the sheets later in the day. Remember: neatness is part of my peace of mind. I kept my room tidy. I thought of it more as a dorm room/living space than a hospital room. I showered and was dressed by 7:00 a.m. before the first doctor entered my room. I wanted to look alert and healthy for the doctors.

If I was not eating, conversing with my team, or working on my computer, I was walking the halls with Ginger, my chemo pole. HCI is in an oval floor design with patient rooms having a view to the outside with beautiful mountain views. Medical stations, the supply center, elevators, and meeting rooms were all in the center of the oval.

One loop in the hallway equaled one-twelfth of a mile, twelve loops to the mile. I told myself, "I CAN do that!" Walking had always been a form of moving meditation and relaxation for me. Because I had always walked a lot, it now signaled my body that I was still functioning; all systems were GO.

I also found that walking got me out and about in my new community into my new "circle of friends." In the first loop, staff would smile and nod. "A patient is out moving. That's good." During the next loop staff would comment to me, "You are looking good." During the third loop, the staff started to give me high fives. During the fourth loop and thereafter, they would laugh, joke, and comment. We developed connections.

Some fellow patients saw me pass their doorway again and again. Some would come out and join me. Several nurses told me that patients would say to them, "I have to walk today. I have to keep up with that guy who is always walking." Staff informally reported that three times as many patients tended to walk if there was a motivated patient on the floor. Others shut their door because they did not want to see me.

I met several new cancer friends during my hallway walks. We instantly became friends with a common bond. My new friends included Brian, Colton, John, and Rand. We all had different stories regarding our cancer diagnoses, but we had a will to fight the disease.

To demonstrate my energy level to the doctors, I walked two miles each morning before my 9:00 daily doctor meeting. I timed the walks and did each mile under twenty minutes. The doctors commented that my walks did indeed help verify my condition and how I felt. I also made sure the doctors saw me walking to show them I was not exaggerating my mileage.

After seven days of chemo, I was eager to start planning to go home. Time had a new meaning.

My short term goals for home

I was not sure how I would weather this period. My goals were modest.

- I love having morning coffee on the deck watching the sunrise on the Utah mountains. I would do this every day.
- We have great Utah sunsets from our front deck. I would relish every one.
- A more forward-thinking goal: Work toward a physical activity that I love. Stay strong to ski. Kathy and I would buy Utah ski passes for the upcoming ski season. I planned to ski on Day 60 after my transplant. To do so, I needed to keep in shape and

work my legs. I could not just lie in bed and expect to be robust during recovery.

- Seven chemo days later, I plan to go home feeling fine. So far, so good!

Fred's Lessons Learned

- I'm not sick. I have a faulty system that needs to be replaced. That's a different psychological message than "I have cancer."
- This is now your community. Meet your fellow patients. We're all in this together. Get out there and mingle. Meet new friends—every patient is like you. They all have stories behind their diagnoses. They were normal people until that phone call came from the doctor with those terrible three words "You have cancer." We met Carol and Jim in the clinic, and we are now good friends. I developed a deep friendship with Brian, Colton, John, Rand, and other transplant patients.
- Meet the staff and get to know them as people—doctors, physician assistants (PAs), nurses, HCAs, cleaning staff—they are all important and want to help. Write down names of aides, nurses, PAs, doctors, and administration staff. There will be a lot of people involved in your journey. I kept track of daily staff in the medical journal.
- You are a key member of your medical team. Stay involved, ask questions, take notes, and have an agenda for each doctor meeting.
- STAY OUT OF BED. Bed is the worst place to be unless there is a true need for a day of rest. One result of staying in bed is that you quickly lose muscle tone and it's difficult to get it back. The bed is not a Barcalounger.
- Exercise. Find an exercise routine that helps your mental state, but you need to find a routine that you will stick with, even when you are feeling lousy. Exercise like your life depends on it, because it does! Full body exercise delivers oxygen to every cell in your body.

- Medical fact tells us that even healthy people, when confided to bed for a week, will lose a great deal of physical strength and bone mass. Your job is to build and maintain strength, because there is more of this road ahead.
- HCI had an excellent Wellness Center with trained staff to assist physical conditioning throughout hospitalization and after being discharged. It also provided a stationary bike for my room at my request.
- Walking. I first kept track of loops with pennies (Kathy washed them beforehand) from my pocket to Ginger's tray. We'd collect the daily accumulation in a jar to see my efforts. I later used a Fitbit to track mileage. I did a minimum of two miles per day and hit seven miles one day! I became Fitbit friends with several of the nurses. A little competition motivated me to do a few more laps.
- Eat healthy. Make good food choices. It's about fueling, not feelings. Be careful what you eat before chemo. Don't eat your favorite foods and ruin future enjoyment by negative association.
- Dress for success. Look normal, feel normal. Stay out of the ugly hospital gowns.
- Hair loss is very likely at some point with chemo.
  - » Shaving your head in advance can be an act of control. I was in control by determining when I would go bald.
  - » For men, there are good looking role models, including Yul Brynner, Bruce Willis, and Mr. Clean.
  - » For women, you can take this opportunity to be wild and crazy with wigs, scarves, and hats.
  - » Bald heads (both men and women) get cold. Find some wild or warm hats to wear for warmth.
- Like the Tim McGraw country western song "Live Like You Were Dying", be in the moment. You have the gift of the day. Don't waste it.
- "Chemo is hell. The only thing worse than chemo is cancer." (Nurse Bob)

Fred's Game Plan

- I am a contributing team member.
- I am a contributing member to my hospital community.
- I am doing all I can to be healthy and strong.
- Recovery is my work. These are not "sick days" to lie around and wait for it to pass. It's onward every day toward the goal. Lack of progression adds to regression. A small step forward is still forward.

Your Game Plan

- How do I spend my time?
- Where can I find space to move?
- How many miles did I walk today?
- How many new friends did I meet outside of my room?
- Did I say "Thank you" to all the staff? They are ALL trying very hard to help me.

Your Medical Journal

- How does this first experience go?
- Start a medical diary of your key blood count numbers, how you feel, medications and what they do, and any issues that advance or recede. It's helpful information. You'll find it a good reference, because you can't count on remembering, as the days blur. Someday your medical journal may be a good reference for someone else.
- It's a good habit to keep track of what you eat and drink with estimated calories and volume. Your body is internally processing at high speed. Your systems need fuel.

Your Internal Journal

Remember the description about stress and mindset? There's "threat mindset" and "challenge mindset." The difference is a tiny pause that permits a choice of staying in basic survival mode or moving to challenge mode. Research says when people name what they are feeling, their brain activity moves to the higher level. Writing decreases emotional response and allows for thought and analysis to return, putting you back in the drivers' seat. By writing you can decrease the raw intensity of emotions by shifting from experiencing emotion to observing them. Writing provides structure. Seeing your words has a power that lets you accept, correct, or control your thinking patterns.

When you feel the grip of emotion, try a tiny pause to breathe and think and then try writing about it. It's your private space. Do something consciously to stop the rush of fear.

Hospital Life
A Prolonged Stay

All of us are stronger than one of us.
Your body, your cancer.....Our fight
- Signed your health team

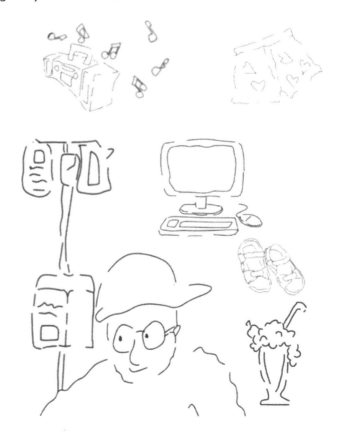

This is my world

For several months, HCI was my world and the staff members were my people.

My goal was to live as normally as I could in this abnormal environment for a stretch of time.

The entire check-in process was surreal. It would have been easy to let the circumstances take control and define the experiences. The staff led me into my room, showed me my bed with a cross-bed table, indicated my hospital gown, and showed me my call button, my bed controls, and my TV remote. It would have been easy just to put on the hospital gown, climb into bed, and turn on the TV—for several months.

Instead I was thinking, "How can I be normal?"

Your hospital room: Make it personal

Kathy and I learned the importance of differentiating our space. There was sleeping space and living space. Our biggest find was a small, adjustable table for the living area used for eating, computer work, and other daytime activities. Otherwise, the only table was the cross-bed table encouraging patients to eat, use their computers and watch TV in bed. We requested that this across-bed table be removed to give me more room as I maneuvered with my pole, "Ginger."

We happened to have a small portable computer table at home. We also found Tablemate, a small adjustable table available at Walmart and Bed, Bath and Beyond. Consider it a good gift to a friend caught in a prolonged hospital stay.

We decorated the living space so that it became a comfortable place to spend time. Kathy sanitized throw pillows to use on the coach and chairs to make them fit comfortably. We brought a radio for music and talk radio. We had Fred Jr., a stuffed bear from a young nephew, and Mini-Melissa, a Care Bear dressed in scrubs from a young niece. (We had five nurses named Melissa at one time.) We had Chico, a plush monkey with his own mountain wardrobe, made by another family member. These collections of goodwill gifts were our in-house cheering team that added fun to the room. It doesn't sound like the somber room of a sixty-two-year-old male.

We brought in decorated boxes to keep loose items controlled, so that the room didn't get messy. Remember, neatness was part of my peace of mind. The room was cheerful, colorful, and uncluttered.

These personal touches gave the staff insight into me as a person as well as a patient. There was always something for discussion. "So, what's with the monkey?"

Clothing

Clean socks and footwear, soft sweat pants, soft T-shirts, polar fleece zip sweaters (temperatures in hospitals are often cold to suppress germs), funny boxer shorts (to lighten up the request where there was the need to drop pants to examine my infected leg), and NO hospital gowns. I had a hat collection. Your head gets cold when you lose your hair. I was glad to have sunglasses so that "Ginger" and I could go out on a terrace when it was shaded. We preferred sun in the room to closed shades; however, the eyes are very sensitive to light during and after chemo.

Footwear is a big deal. Fall for any reason, and hospital life gets very complicated. You become a "fall risk." Wear flimsy or slippery footwear and risk being stuck in bed for safety reasons. Think twice about walking around in socks, athletic slides, flip-flops, and bedroom slippers. Clean sneakers worked fine. My best choice was athletic Keen sandals. They secured to my foot with Velcro straps. They were comfortable with or without socks. They could be washed and kept clean.

More about exercise—it's that big of a deal!

Moving by my own power reminded me that I was still strong enough to navigate on my own. I felt it was important to keep my muscles working and my lungs and heart pumping. Oxygen is a critical element to be delivered to all my cells. AML is a problem of inefficient red blood cells not delivering oxygen to my body. Lie around, and the lungs breathe shallowly and create small, moist seams at the edges where bacteria can breed. Stand upright, and the lungs are held open. A common risk is opportunistic pneumonia, so you need to keep your lungs open, moving, and strong; all systems GO.

Friends from India lovingly talked about the power of breath and gave us instructions on mindful breathing. There are many studies about the impact deep breathing has on the involuntary systems. Deep breathing is something you can do that's easy and has significant benefits. I include a more detailed discussion and a website link in the Resource and Reference section.

Just get moving one step at a time. Feel the rhythm and the flow. It's an accomplishment. It's a normal activity. It's something I could do. It became part of my stress management. It became part of my socialization. I shared positive energy with other patients. "Hey, we're moving! We're working! Today we're doing OK." Ginger and I received positive energy from the staff.

Food

I had a calorie and liquid intake requirement. If I managed it myself, I could go home.

Eating and drinking is worth noting. There are times when you will have no appetite or when food and liquids are repulsive. Intravenous (IV) nutrition is not an easy default food and liquid replacement. It is a serious consideration and often a last resort. It is important to keep your digestive tract active and functioning. You will need to figure out ways to eat and drink a required amount each day. If you can't eat and drink independently, you stay in the hospital longer. I learned to track my own calories and liquids reliably in my medical journal. Staff might get busy and forget to record small items. I double checked the end-of-day tally. There were times when each ounce counted toward my going home.

Quick story: The Linda Special. One day nothing sounded good to eat, but I had a minimum calorie goal. I also wanted the intake to be relatively healthy. It's a cross between requirement, comfort food, and nutrition. I chose a plain veggie burger with no bun and some chips. Linda, a friendly food delivery staff member, happened to see my name on this wimpy meal and asked for this delivery assignment. The pleasant little woman marched into my room with a bee in her bonnet. She informed me that my choice was not a good lunch and reminded me I needed a combination of calories and nutrients. She suggested I order a breakfast protein shake made with ice cream for added calories. It's cold. It's wet. It's pleasant tasting, with a choice of flavors. It has some nutrition to it. It slides down easily as little sips through a straw. It might take me three hours to get it down, but I managed it and registered 600 calories (my daily calorie requirement was 1,500 calories).

My comfort food was yogurt. Like the Linda Special, it is cold and wet and slides down. It has a variety of flavors. The hospital choice was a no-fat, no-sugar, low-calorie, and no-taste variety. Kathy brought a full-fat Greek fruit yogurt. On a good day, I could get two or three of those down to help me get to my daily calorie requirement. Eventually we noticed that I wasn't having as many stomach problems as we observed in other patients. (Remember: "Every body is unique. Every body is a mystery.") We wondered if the yogurt was cultivating the good bacteria in my stomach as chemo was scrambling the balance in my digestive system. Perhaps yogurt was just soothing to my system. (Caution: Yogurt during chemo cannot contain probiotics, because probiotics include active bacteria. Ask the hospital nutritionist before eating yogurt purchased from outside the hospital.)

In praise of Angel Mints: These specialty mints contain four basic ingredients including oil of peppermint. Many patients report that these mints soothe nausea. I still keep them around for the occasional upset stomach. They also offset the metallic task that lingers from some medications. Many hospital giftshops carry them. They can be acquired online from www.AngelMint.com.

Hygiene

You will read about the ever-present world of bacteria and viruses in us and around us. EVERYONE uses hand sanitizer as he/she enters and exits every patient room. With compromised immune systems, good hygiene is critical.

Soapy showers every day was a requirement. Bacteria live on our skin. Clean clothes are also a necessity.

Consider a new, clean, soft toothbrush or a soft electric toothbrush for thorough, gentle oral hygiene. "Swish and Spit" is a quick rinse of salt, baking soda, and water. Get in the habit of using that technique every time you are in the bathroom.

Addressing Time: It's a waiting game for results

Am I bored because I'm sick? Do I feel sick because I'm bored? Am I really bored, or am I depressed? If I'm bored, I can do something about it. If I'm depressed, I don't have the energy to do anything about it and need assistance. Call it like it is, and do what needs to be done. Get a plan of action or a plan of assistance. It's a tough road. Don't make it tougher.

Studies show that people who intentionally created conditions in their day that were likely to bring about positive emotions have more happy feelings and fewer symptoms of depression than those who didn't. Take charge and create positive conditions in your day. Look for ways to add activities that are pleasing. Don't expect rip-roaring fun, but have reasonable expectations to enjoy the moment. Take wonder in the small things, because you are there to behold them. Be in the moment. Know up front that you will be interrupted regularly, and go with the flow.

The Art of Conversation

Appreciate your team of the day, your hospital care staff. "So, Nurse Matt, how did you end up here? Have you always wanted to be in medicine? What did you want to be when you were a little kid? What do you want to be when you were a little kid? What do you do in your off hours that balances the stress of this work? What's your story?"

(Matt's story: He is a survivor of brain cancer and became a nurse. He is a remarkable man and a very cool guy.)

Seeing University of Michigan paraphernalia in the room, a Chinese-American nurse shared her father's story of being a foreign engineering student at the University of Michigan pre-World War II, returning to his homeland as an engineer during wartime and later being caught in the Chinese Cultural Revolution. This story was fascinating and an experience to hear! We learned the stories and aspirations of the medical workers from other countries who've come with extraordinary experiences. These exceptional people populate this difficult medical world.

Listen to good conversation: talk radio works as a good stimulus sometimes. It can be interesting, fresh conversation about the outside world. Other times, it can be annoying chatter with reminders of an aggressive world. Keep politics out of this arena. Everyone's blood pressure readings need to stay low.

Reading

Medications can fuzz up vision, mental focus, and retention.

On good days, reading is the opportunity to escape the physical world and transport to another time, place, and space through the power of books. Haven't learned the value and pleasure of books? This is your chance. Be an optimist and relish this opportunity to mentally escape, seek adventure, and explore. Audio books can equally whisk you away through good storytelling. Feed your brain good ideas as your body mends and heals.

Audio books are sometimes lengthy, however, and may not be the best choice for drowsy days. Ted Talks are short, informative, stimulating, and less than twenty minutes long. Talk radio (PBS and NPR) provided a wide range of life topics. Podcasts are specific discussions for your selections. Learn something new. Have something interesting to share and communicate. Be an interested, interesting patient. If you don't have these resources readily available, ask the hospital activity person or contact the teens in your family. Chances are they have them all!

All this reading and listening loops back to the art of conversation: good input/good output. Find an interesting thought for the day and ask the opinion of staff members as they come to do routine tasks. Get outside yourself.

Music

Controlled music comes in many forms: MP3 player, iPod, or clock radio with disc player and CDs. Listening to music can boost your brainpower, but only if you tune in to happy songs.

Many studies report that people respond more quickly when uplifting tunes were played during testing. Upbeat, not necessarily fast-paced songs may produce dopamine, a neurotransmitter that improves working memory, resulting in a sharper, more focused mind. We think it fills the room with energy rather than silence broken by the hiss, squeak, and beep of medical equipment. It's energizing and a change of pace for staff members who often commented how nice it was to have music in the room.

Movies

We did not make time for movies, but movie selection should probably follow the same guidelines for positive, upbeat, dopamine-producing effect. There's enough scary stuff happening in your world. You don't need to be importing any more stress.

Television

Television is a habit. It fills the air with rapid, fast-paced sounds and pictures. The flow of stories and information is regularly interrupted by commercials, many of which are built on principles of annoyance as a memory tool. The more this medium is on, the less effective it is in keeping us stimulated. It can become meaningless noise that distracts us from other activities.

Keep it special. Use it wisely. Kathy and I watched only special events for entertainment. If/when eating became a challenge, I would need a distraction from the menacing food on the fork. We would find something interesting on TV or video and I could eat somewhat mindlessly.

Mix it up

On a good day, tackle activities that challenge. The body might be creaking, but the mind can still zing! Try puzzles, word games, and mazes. Make plans! Research projects for your time ahead. We did the research and prepared to buy a new car for future adventures when all this medical stuff was over.

Use the day to give as well as receive. Write notes to others, rather than just receiving messages from others. Make Valentines of appreciation, no matter what time of year. Tell your story via written or recorded journaling. Use this gift of time. It's the present. We now understand time is a limited commodity.

If this scare has given you pause for thought about your relationships, perhaps this time is the time to connect with clarity. Two books are noted below that we found helped structure our thinking and our written conversation. Like the journal, this area is private and under your control. Work on it for your benefit. Decide if, when, and how you'd like to share it or not. Decide how you will use this time.

A Conversation with My Children: A Guided Journal for Parents to Share their Story & Heart with Their Adult Children by Terrika Faciane

> "This guided journal will be a place to let your life speak; to leave a living legacy for your children and grandchildren. Your story matters; and no one can share it better than you."

Memories for My Child by Peter Pauper Press

"Record details of your life, family history, values, memories, and more for your children by following the prompts in this appealing keepsake journal."

See the Resource and Reference section in the back of this book for more details on these two publications.

Communicating to family and friends: Your philosophy

Correspondence was important work for us and an important part of each day. Every day new e-mails would arrive and would generate lots of conversation. We felt supported, energized, and loved by this direct, personal contact.

It started with phone calls and a few e-mails to immediate family and close friends and eventually expanded to more than 200 people around the world. People want to know what's happening. If they didn't hear within a week, they started to worry, expecting bad news. Rather than use an efficient social-media service, we wrote a general e-mail as a progress report once a week and sent it out as a group e-mail. People replied, and we responded. We found that the individual e-mails were a high point each day. Other patients used CaringBridge or Facebook.

Quick story: One nurse gave me the title Mayor of the Fourth Floor because of my high visibility. One day staff and visitors came from 9:00 a.m. until 4:00 p.m., almost nonstop. I groused to Kathy that I couldn't get to my e-mails and it was backing up. Her quick reply was, "Well, that's what you get for being the mayor of the fourth floor!" Point made! I appreciate the caring of the many friends I have made within this hospital community.

Know that some days will be riddled with interruptions. Go with the flow.

Your Internal Journal

When we tell the story of our experience, we create a coherent, consistent narrative about it. The swirling inside takes shape, can be named and examined. It can take the form of letters to yourself, letters to others, letters to God, letters to cancer. And it's all private.

"(Adversity) made me a writer. When something (bad) happens or it happened to me, I wanted to be the one who was telling the story instead of the one it was happening to. ´ - Jennifer Weiner

Life At Home After Chemo

May you live every day of your life.
- Jonathan Swift

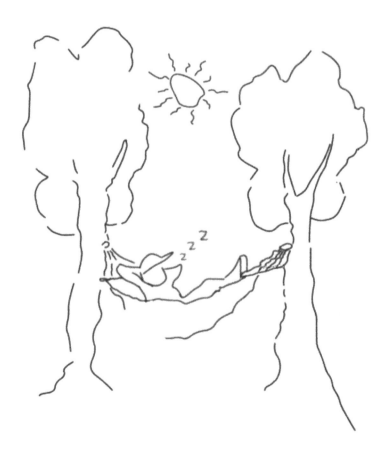

Home after Seven Days of Chemo–Yay!

WOW! I made it through the initial seven days of heavy duty chemo with minimal side effects, good energy, and an optimistic outlook. I was still alive and the doctors were going to let me go home! Home sweet home! There is indeed NO PLACE LIKE HOME! In my own bed without my "vitals" being taken at midnight and 4:00 a.m., I could get a full night sleep.

The doctors decided to discharge me after seven days of chemo because I was doing so well. The plan was to observe me for three more weeks. However, instead of being observed in the hospital, I could visit an outpatient clinic every other day.

The primary concern was a fever since my immune system had been shut down by the chemo. There was a 50/50 probability that I would need to return to the hospital to deal with a fever and some type of infection.

The other concerns were how well the chemo destroyed all the bad leukemia cells. Whether my blood cells were doing what they should be doing. Most likely I would need to return for more chemo.

Kathy and I needed a new routine for home

Walking was part of the plan. I was clocking miles at the hospital. We lived at the top of a steep hill. Could I manage the exertion? We decided to try driving and parking at a neighboring street at the bottom of the hill. We walked along the level street several times. Kathy left me under the shade of a tree to get the parked car. As she swung by to pick me up at the bottom of the hill, she got nervous when I wasn't there. As she started up the hill in the car, she found me waiting at the top of the steep hill. It felt great to be able to tackle that challenging task.

Stairs were also part of the plan. We live in a condo. I worked my way to twenty-two flights of ascending stairs. My goal was to ski. It requires leg strength. I worked toward my goal.

My infusion PICC line

PICC Line: Peripherally Inserted Central Catheter, a form of intra-venous access that can be used for a prolonged period of time.

Hail to the visiting nurse services. Pat and her colleagues were on call 24/7. Pat came on the day of release to do several things. She instructed us on how to maintain the hygiene of my PICC infusion lines and any home infusion medication. (YouTube will also demo it for you, but the nurses are available anytime help is needed.) She quietly observed the hygiene of the home and discussed good home practices, which boiled down to clean, clean, clean. She kept track of home medical supplies and replenished as expected. She or her colleagues visited us between clinic visits to confirm all was well.

At first this PICC line responsibility was daunting. It took two of us to navigate the steps and manage the materials. It soon became routine. After a bit of time I was able to care for this task myself.

Eating at home

We had control over our diet. We are both of small stature, which means we have to eat carefully. Our friend Peter coached us on increasing our attention to nutrition. First we found that in order to eat fresh fruits and vegetables, we needed to clean and sanitize them, get the dirt off; get the germs off. Keep the nutrients in. Peter convinced us that juicing fruits and vegetables was our most efficient way of getting the biggest impact from the power of food. Since it was farmer's market season, lots of produce was readily available.

We washed, sanitized, juiced, and then cleaned the juicing machine. It was approximately an hour's worth of work for eight ounces of icky green juice. We strived for maximum nutrition from the most powerful greens we could find with less regard for taste. I managed to get the smoothies down when accompanied by a slice of multigrain bread. Interestingly, after five days of this regimen, we both noticed that our skin was glowing. You are what you eat.

Sanitizing

Fresh fruits and vegetables need special care to be sure they are free of dirt and germs from growing and handling. Rinsing with water doesn't do the job. We chose to purchase an ozonating machine. Kathy washed the produce, soaked it in ozonated water for a few minutes, and then continued preparation.

Kathy also sprayed the processed water on soft items, such as throw pillows to be used in my hospital room. She would do a quick spray through the house at night to clean the kitchen, baths, knobs, and soft furniture, in an attempt to clean without chemicals.

Fred's Lessons Learned

- Exercising made me feel that I had strength and was capable. Climbing the hill was a reassurance that I was not deteriorating.
- I had an IV treatment that I could do at home. It was clever technology that was convenient. We just needed to learn how to do it with the vigilant care required.
- Juicing was tolerable. I was willing to do it if it advanced my efforts to be healthy.
- Watch your comfort foods. Sure, you've lost weight and your body's working hard. Sugar consumption lessens our ability to fight off infections. The process of white blood cells engulfing virus and bacteria is significantly reduced when you eat simple sugars. Use sugars carefully to accomplish a goal like ice cream in the Linda Special.

During the initial seven days of chemo, we realized the importance of establishing goals and having the meaning of life in front of us.

Here were our initial goals. They may seem trivial, but after seven days of chemo, they are suddenly VERY significant. Put into perspective, chemo creates a realization of the miracle of life.

- Make it through seven days of chemo.
- Return home.
- Enjoy sunrises and sunsets from our condo deck.
- Take a walk together.
- Enjoy uninterrupted sleep in my own bed.

I learned that Johnny Runner, my hospital buddy, was back to light hiking and training. I realized my aspirations were too low. I picked up my activities to a more normal pace. Don't convince yourself you are infirm when you still have energy. John became a role model and benchmark for me. He helped me see more potential in myself.

Communicating with friends and family

- Keep communicating on a frequent basis. People DO want to hear from you. Be honest in what's happening and how you are feeling, but end the communication with a positive statement of your fight.
- No news is bad news. Stay in touch.
- Our friend Charles stated in his e-mail, "No matter how you look at this situation, it really sucks!" This e-mail was the most honest, straightforward one received from our friends and family.
- Be honest with others but stay positive. "Bad day today, but I'm ready for better things tomorrow."
- Be proactive in your relationships with others. They are also scared and not sure how to interact with you.
- Be up front and honest in telling others about your situation: "I have cancer, and I'm in the fight. GAME ON."
- Communicate—e-mail, blogs, Facebook, CaringBridge; do SOMETHING on a regular basis.
  - » Our chosen communication method—e-mail, instead of blogging or Facebook
    - ▪ Blogs: Family and friends have to take the initiative to look at your blog.
    - ▪ Facebook: Not everyone is on Facebook.

» Our method: "Fred Update" e-mails. Recipients knew from the e-mail subject line there was a significant event. Our distribution list started at fifteen people and expanded to more than 200 as friends heard and asked to be kept informed.

» We responded to everyone who replied to our e-mails. If they took the time to connect, then I needed to take the time to acknowledge, even if it is just a quick "Thanks for your note."

» We had periodic phone discussions so people could hear my voice. I could fake being OK in an e-mail, but I can't fake it on the telephone.

» Phone calls can take up a lot of time and are necessary; however, we found electronic communications to be more efficient.

Your Internal Journal

"How can I know what I think until I see what I say?"
– E.M. Foster

Focused
Philosophy

Once you choose HOPE, anything is possible.
- Christopher Reeve

No disease likes hope.
- Hindi proverb

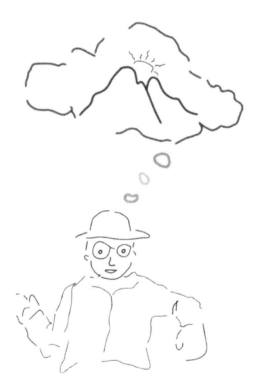

Signature phrases to keep the focus

Chardi Kala!

Our good friends, the Gills, are Sikhs. We received a package of two soft cotton T-shirts with Chardi Kala embroidered on the fronts. (char DEEK ala...sounds like a happy chirp.)

They explained to us that Chardi Kala is a core concept for Sikhs. It refers to a mental state of optimism and joy. These Punjabi words can be translated as "positive attitude" or "ascending energy." The term is also described as being in "high spirits" or a "positive, buoyant, and optimistic" attitude to life and to the future.

Chardi Kala is "the state of mind in which a person has no negative emotions like fear or jealousy. Instead the mind is full of positive feelings including joy, satisfaction, and self-dignity based on their belief in a merciful God. This allows one to face hardships and to help others in their hour of need." (Source: SikhiWiki)

In history, it was a powerful psychological weapon used by Sikhs to fight armies that vastly outnumbered them. In the cancer world, every patient and their families need a powerful psychological weapon, because the threat feels overwhelming.

We had a sense of the needed effort. The Chardi Kala philosophy immediately resonated with us. It started us thinking on a clearer path. It gave us a common language to discuss what we needed in terms of reaching for inner strength. It became a guiding philosophy with clear language and powerful feeling. Without a clear alternative, the default feeling was fear.

Keep a positive, uplifting, and optimistic attitude to life and to the future!

Positive: Positivity is not just a way of thinking. It's a way of feeling at the moment. It's an effort as well as an intention. It's giving your best. It's doing all you can do.

Uplifting: Feeling uplifted is a vision and understanding at a high level. It's pride in action.

Optimistic attitude to life and to the future: Chardi Kala is about honing the meaning of life.

In the cancer experience, Chardi Kala is the conversation you need to hear. Although the medical staff was kind and loving, they communicated with a needed level of science and technicality. They could not deliver a warrior's message when treatment was uncertain. When applicable, their messaging, as required by law, was about possible side effects that sometimes included the words "and can be fatal," to cover all the bases. These stated realities did not encourage or empower us.

Chardi Kala became our battle cry, our mantra, our closing in our communication with family and friends. It became our standard reflection at the end of each day, generally concluding, "Today was actually fun." Chardi Kala in action!

Quick story: Staff members regularly told us that my good effort was the exception, not the norm. As a result, I regularly received profuse kudos from the nursing staff, usually young professional females who kept telling me that I was doing awesome or I looked awesome. I LOVED it and we laughed at the frequency.

I walked, ate, and connected (positive effort). Staff members told me that I was awesome (positive shared feelings). I worked harder because I had an "awesome" reputation to maintain (uplifting). The staff was more impressed (uplifting). My efforts brought me closer to a good outcome. My future was closer to being realized. Chardi Kala!

Awesome adulations went on regularly for the first two years (daily during the hospital stay and clinic visits thereafter). Over time staff turned over. One day we passed through the patient floor and I said to Kathy, "No one has said I looked awesome." Within fifteen seconds Ryan, a big, burly male physical therapist, rounded the corner. In his booming voice, he shouted, "Hey, Fred. You look awesome!" and gave me a crushing bear hug. It was not quite the thrill of doting young female attention, but I appreciated it just the same.

We made cards with the Chardi Kala message as a way of sharing this powerful philosophy. We thanked our Sikh friends and their culture for maintaining the power of this message throughout the ages and keeping it vibrant for today's challenges.

Game On!

A friend ended his good-wishes e-mail to us with a rousing "**Game on.**" Another score! We knew the only hope was a successful outcome to the transplant. Trying to wish it away, dreading the event, or hoping for a miracle wasn't going to accomplish anything.

Game on. Welcome the new stem cells. Invite them to move in and make a happy home. We encouraged the existing cells to make friends and play nice, as these newcomers would bring prospects of good life.

Internal Journal

What's going to be your philosophy to get you moving forward?

What's your self-talk? What are you telling yourself?

Be still and quiet and listen to the talk that surfaces from within. Are these the messages that you want to take you to your desired end? Are you sending a positive message to your new self?

Setbacks And Unexpected Challenges

It's all unexpected!

Just when you think it can't get any worse, it can.
And just when you think it can't get any better, it can.
- Nicholas Sparks

Courage doesn't always roar.
Sometimes courage is the quiet voice at the end of the day, saying,
"I will try again tomorrow."
- Mary Anne Radmacher

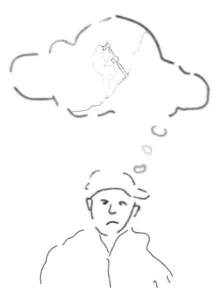

Unexpected challenges should be expected. There are things you can control. There are things you can influence. There are things you can't control.

Problems: Back at the hospital as inpatient

The first week at home after seven days of chemo was great. I then started feeling sluggish and I could feel my temperature rising, despite a normal thermometer reading. Listen to your body. I knew I had a temperature, but the thermometer did not indicate any. We decided to be proactive and head to the outpatient clinic to get a doctor's opinion. While I was at the clinic my temperature soared. We all agreed that I was back as inpatient for another stay.

I didn't catch something at home. I had it with me all along. We are not alone in our bodies. We have exposure to many virus and bacteria from the larger world that resides within our bodies. Our healthy systems keep bugs in check. Without the immune system humming away, unusual things often blossom and bloom and baffle the medical staff. Finding the right remedy often is trial and error. Remember, every body is unique. Every body is a mystery.

The other not-so-good news was the result of my bone marrow biopsy. The bone marrow biopsy sounds scary, but it was tolerable. Yup, they do indeed puncture your hip with a big needle. The bone marrow biopsy showed the chemo worked effectively but 10% of the bad guys were still in my system, which required five more days of chemo. Since I was back as an inpatient fighting the bacteria, the decision was to be efficient and multitask with chemo.

More bad news. I had a little red bump on my leg that became inflamed. Within days I had a huge swollen, blackening leg that was not responding to the various antibiotic treatments. My left thigh was two to three times larger than the right thigh. The concern was that this infection would sink into the muscle, filter into my blood system, and be fatal.

The team of professionals grew as the medical personnel brought in new specialists to add insight. The surgeons were buzzing around to remove infected tissue if needed. The doctors gave it everything they had and admitted that they did not know what else to do.

I said to my doctor, "It looks like you are giving me every type of antibiotic."

The doctor replied, "We are and we hope one of them starts working."

One morning my leg suddenly looked better, to the doctors' amazement. The doctor comments included, "Hey, I think it looks better!" "I think so, too!" and "Thank you, God!" Your body does repair work overnight. I had dodged another bullet.

A weird lung condition (San Joaquin Valley Fever) developed. The infectious disease team indicated that I had likely acquired it from hiking in the Arizona desert on a vacation in the past. The Utah Department of Health contacted me to track my treatment progress, because San Joaquin Valley Fever is rare in Utah.

I had opportunistic pneumonia twice. While never debilitating, it required treatment. I had my share of strange stuff. I slugged through all of it. All of these problems occurred because my immune system had shut down.

One other news item: The official bone marrow donor search started. The only option to cure my problem was a bone marrow transplant. The search was on for someone with a ten-by-ten match with my DNA. We wondered where the person would come from, most likely from the USA or Europe. Would it be male or female? Female stem cells are an option! WOW! This modern medicine is amazing!

Five Weeks as an Inpatient

Before my diagnosis, I had never spent a night in a hospital. After my diagnosis I was an inpatient for seven days with a projected four to five additional weeks. BOO!

The stay was not too bad. I had a routine. I exercised often, and I made new friends. There are two types of friends: friends and cancer friends (fellow patients). There is no closer bond than that which is shared with cancer friends, and only members of the cancer club are invited into that friendship.

Luckily during my month as an inpatient, the Summer Olympics took place, so I was able to watch a lot of the Olympic events. I saw much more of the Olympics than if I were a "regular" person at home.

Many of the staff members were runners or mountain bikers, so they were interested in watching the Olympics but could not, while working, so we worked a deal. The nurses would tell me what events they wanted to watch. I would press the Patient Assist button, and the appropriate nurse would come to "assist" me and watch his or her event. I received a LOT of special care during the Olympic games! For the men's 100 meter finals I had a room full of nurses to see the ten-second event.

The hospital was like my second home. I received frequent hugs and good wishes from the staff. Ryan, a new male nurse, introduced himself to me one day. He wanted to meet "Fred." He said the nurses and aides were all fighting over who would work with me, probably because I tried to be low maintenance.

Phase one was completed. Good news regarding the chemo: Seven days of chemo followed by five days of more chemo killed the bad cells for the desired results, and I was now "squeaky clean." My concern was that my ANC count was at zero for a month and thus I had no immune system to fight off the bad things inside me. I was getting nervous. What if the ANC never started moving up?

ANC is an important number. Absolute Neutrophil Count is a calculation of white blood cell factors that measure a person's infection fighting ability. At ANC=0 you have no immune system, and bad things can easily happen. With ANC at 500, there is generally sufficient protection to fend off the risks of being home. Normal is 1500 to 8000/mm3.

As we watched my ANC count, I was in training for the transplant. I worked with a physical trainer to help me get in the best condition in terms of weight and condition. He conducted research on cancer and physical conditioning. He was convinced there was a direct correlation between physical conditioning and the probability of a successful treatment; hence he provided more encouragement to keep doing the workouts.

I mapped out walking routes that exceeded my previous paths. Doctors were dismayed at my initial plans to hike to the nearby arboretum, and they kept me on the hospital grounds. I found walking was a forward-moving skill. Climbing stairs was dramatically harder. There were approximately 125 ascending steps around the building. When I could be separated from "Ginger" for a portion of the day, I worked my way up to eight round trips for 1,000 ascending steps.

After I spent thirty-two days as an inpatient, the ANCs hit their mark and exceeded 500. With great effort I was eating and drinking according to the requirements. I was on my way home.

Donors Are Backing Out—Schedule Delays

Good news—at least twenty potential donors had been identified that had a ten-by-ten match with my DNA. The match program selected a specific person to be my donor. YES! Let's get on with the transplant!

Some things you can't control. We were scheduled to start the stem cell process in mid-October. Unfortunately, a week prior to the start of the preparation procedures, the donor opted out. It would take four to six weeks to go through the donor investigation process again. The odds of leukemia cells returning in the next few weeks were high; therefore the standard process is more chemo. I was back as inpatient to start the same chemo process that I had done twice before. It once again knocked my blood cell counts and ANCs to zero, with the same risks resulting from no immune system. Bummer!

We were taking this process one step at a time and one day at a time, as reminded by my good friend Joel. The donor's action of backing out was obviously very disappointing, because I was physically and mentally ready for the next phase. Kathy and I concluded that we simply needed to tackle the problem just as we had the others problems we had faced. I would use the time to continue to prepare by building my health. It was more exercise and good nutrition.

During the next two months more discouraging donor news kept arriving. Ten confirmed donors opted to decline when asked to donate. Fortunately I had a common DNA with many potential donors, but time was an issue. Kathy continued to remind me that I was very lucky, that this setback was simply a scheduling delay, and that I needed to continue focusing on staying healthy and in good physical condition. I needed to stay positive, even with the ongoing series of donor disappointments. It was just a matter of finding someone who would follow through on his or her commitment.

I was still using my time to train diligently, but it was protocol to add another round of chemo. A new health issue developed that dealt with a nodule discovered in my lung, based on a chest x-ray.

Once the doctors discovered the lung infection, the constant question I was asked centered on fatigue or difficulty breathing. To demonstrate I was OK, each day I did 1,000 stairs up, without any fatigue or breathing problems. The lung doctors then started calling me their 1,000-stair patient.

Another donor disappointment. My eleventh confirmed donor backed out. My doctors did not want me to get burned again with another extended six- to eight-week delay. They declared an emergency with the Be the Match donor organization, in order to expedite contacting an additional donor. Thank goodness the new donor agreed to go to his hospital immediately for more tests. All the tests went well and he agreed to proceed.

The new potential donor was my twelfth confirmed donor. I hoped he or she kept the faith. Interesting that donor number twelve agreed to proceed on 12/12/12. Clearly twelve was my lucky number. Thank you, number twelve!

Know that staff connects deeply with patients and their struggles. Staff members are a committed team beyond their job titles. Nurse Aime, who we think is the happiest person in the world, pulled me aside before I met with the doctors. She became very serious and teared up.

This was not good, because she was always smiling. Something had to be wrong. She knew that I had some potential serious showstoppers. She said that she dedicated a candle to me at her church and said a special prayer for me after our last meeting. We hugged, and I said it worked, because all my issues suddenly cleared up. She is a very special person!

Back Home as We Prepared for the Transplant

I had frequent outpatient clinic visits with doctor examinations as we planned for the bone marrow transplant, but I was home and enjoying every minute.

To celebrate our first day home, we went to the Utah ski resorts to purchase our season ski passes for the upcoming season. Plan ahead and have a goal. We planned to spend a lot of time on the slopes. We would not let leukemia keep us from skiing. It was a gorgeous Utah day for spending time in the mountains.

We were also back to gentle hiking in the Utah mountains and loving every step.

A few days prior to my leukemia diagnosis, I had climbed to Catherine's Pass, a beautiful mountain pass at 10,000 feet at the Alta Ski Resort. Once the bad news arrived, Kathy and I established specific goals that we wanted to achieve. One key goal was to get back to the top of Catherine's Pass. We did it just a few weeks after I spent more than a month as an inpatient undergoing chemo treatment!

It was a beautiful, blue-sky Utah day and perfect for hiking in the mountains. We still had a rocky, risky road ahead of us, with more chemo in my future as well as a stem cell transplant. However, we were on a mountain peak on a glorious Utah day!

Up to that date I had spent thirty-nine days as an inpatient, endured twelve days of chemo, and overcame three serious infections resulting from having no immune system. I came out of it healthy and back to my fighting weight after losing fifteen pounds.

We were ready for the next phase. We wanted to get this experience behind us and get back to our normal lives.

Fred's Lessons Learned

- Accept that there will be setbacks. Stay hopeful and optimistic in spite of bad news that develops.
- You are what you eat. In the hospital you already have foreign chemicals zipping through your systems. Stress adds its own brand of bad stuff. Add sugar and fat, and you ask your body to take on another major task of processing more unnatural compounds (junk food) and getting it out of you. Give your body a break. Make good food choices.
- Bulk up before the transplant, because you will lose a lot of weight. I lost fifteen pounds during chemo and bulked up to ten pounds overweight before the transplant. I lost twenty-five pounds in the five weeks after the transplant.
- Follow your doctors' advice. Their job is to keep you alive.
- Doctor meetings will often be delayed because they are taking the time necessary for each patient. Stay calm and tolerant.
- Listen to your body; you will learn a lot.

Fred's Game Plan

- "I have places to go, things to do, people to meet." I had goals for each day.
- I worked on cardio endurance by walking and climbing stairs. I worked with weights to maintain muscle tone and strength. I tried to be in the best shape I could, given the gift of extra time and circumstances.
- I drank extra protein shakes for nutrients and calories. I ate fruits and vegetables, because they would be off-limits when my immune system was shut down.
- I tried to find compelling entertainment that would intrigue me, so I would use the time well.

Your Internal Journal

- Dr. Ira Progoff, a noted psychotherapist for Holocaust survivors, found that the clients who wrote in some form of journal were able to work through issues more rapidly.
- Progoff started his clients with expressive writing. Just write without stopping for three minutes, five minutes, until your ideas surface.
- If you haven't tried your internal journal, there's value in starting now.

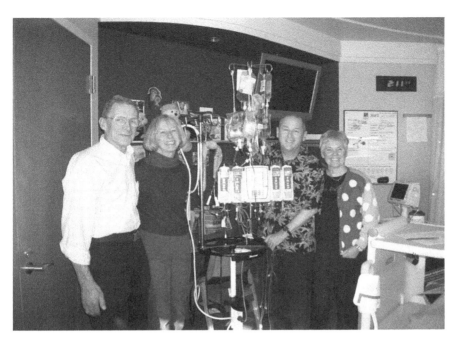

First Transplant
Cousin Bob and wife Sue attending Fred's first stem cell transplant.
Notice Fred's Hawaiian shirt for the Day 0 celebration

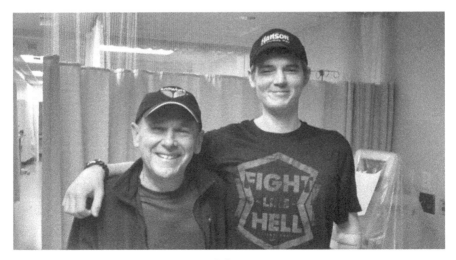

Colton
Nineteen year old Colton and Fred had transplants two days apart.
They became cancer "brothers" and good friends.

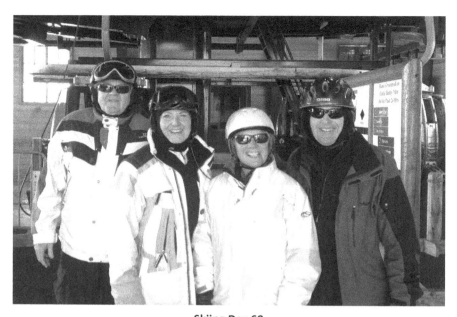

Skiing Day 60
Skiing with friends Jerry and Claudia on Day 60 after the transplant at Deer Valley.
The doctors discouraged skiing so soon after the transplant but it was a huge
moral victory to be on the slopes.

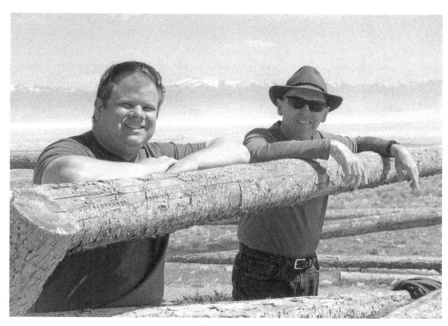

Chris & Fred
Donor Chris and Fred on Antelope Island in the Great Salt Lake. Chris came to
Utah to visit the Huntsman Cancer Institute.

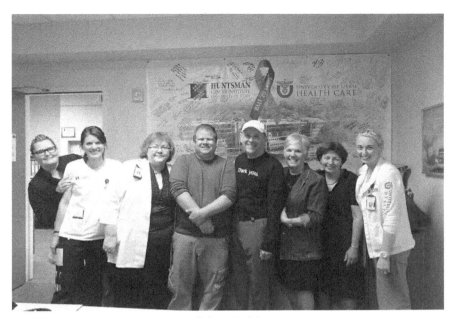

Chris HCI Visit
Donor Chris wanted to see the Huntsman facilities. Chris was treated as a hero during the visit and met over 50 managers and staff.

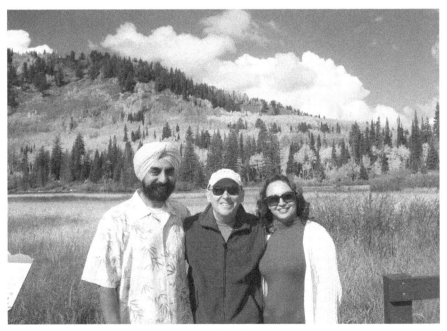

Jasvir & Kaval – Chardi Kala Mentors
Our good friends, Jasvir and Kaval introduced us to the Sikh Chardi Kala philosophy.

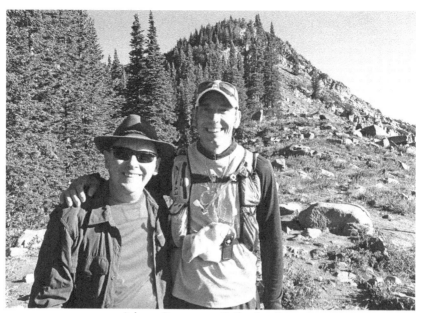

Johnny Runner on Catherine Pass
Johnny Runner (nickname), a fellow transplant patient, runs 100 mile ultra-mountain marathons and was a role model for Fred's recovery strategy. The picture was taken at the top of Catherine Pass.

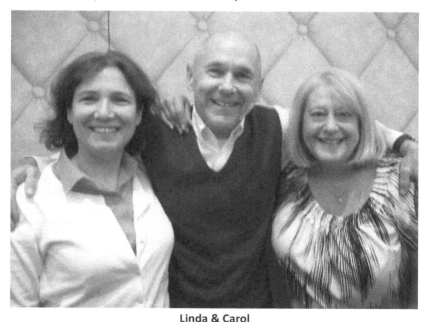

Linda & Carol
Linda and Carol were instrumental in keeping Fred's career alive for the 12 months from his diagnosis to returning to working. We will never be able to adequately express our appreciation!

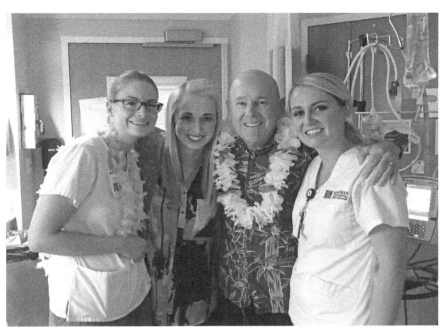

Second Transplant – HCI Staff
The Huntsman nurses involved in Fred's second stem cell transplant.
Hawaiian shirts are Fred's lucky charm.

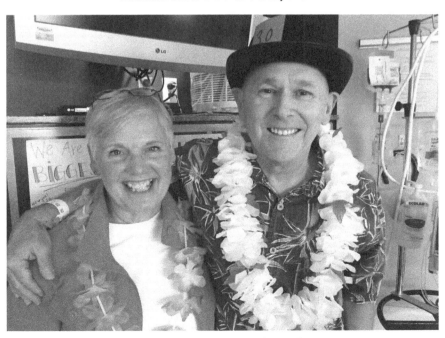

Second Transplant – Fred & Kathy
Fred & Kathy at the second stem cell transplant. We were very hopeful for the future!

Donors—
The Life Savers

DONOR PERSPECTIVES BEFORE THE TRANSPLANT

Written by Chris, our donor

I do it because I can.
- Chris

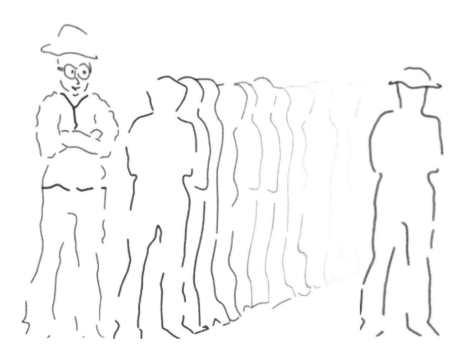

What's the Motivation?

I come from a family of healthy males. My great-great grandfather died not long before my birth (I'm currently twenty-nine years old). I have a vital, vigorous great-grandfather in his nineties. My father is my health role model. I have been aware that my dad gave blood ever since I was young. To me, it was something that men do. I started to go with him, then to donate when I was old enough to participate. It was a special manly outing for us. We started to donate platelets, a three-hour process, when we realized the critical need for them. It was a time to share and talk. Sharing good health is something that we can do

We had a family friend who had leukemia and did not survive, so donating bone marrow, platelets, and blood had always been on my mind. Donating bone marrow is harder. There are fewer donors. It has a short shelf life. Hence, there is an ongoing need from dedicated donors.

As a young male, I decided the next step of involvement was to be a stem cell donor. It involved a mouth swab and a packet of donor information that explained the choices in the process.

Each year the registry sent a letter of recommitment and an update of contact information. One might never be called. It was five years before I received an inquiry. Some people may never be a match.

When I was contacted by Be the Match, I was ready to participate. I was already comfortable with the donation process. I had made the commitment, was healthy, and was willing to follow through.

The Donation Process

I was contacted by Be the Match as a potential match for a patient with need. It requested a preliminary blood workup done locally to confirm general good health and assess more detailed matching. The testing was done at no cost to me. The kit was shipped directly to me. I took it to a local lab, and it sent the kit back to the registry.

I was next contacted two months later indicating I was *the* match for a recipient, and time was very much of the essence. Be the Match Foundation was blunt in expressing that if I didn't donate, the recipient would likely die. The foundation didn't say these things in a threatening or coercing way, more of a matter-of-fact way. I appreciated the frankness.

There was an urgency expressed by Be the Match. Would I be available for a physical exam the next day and a scheduled harvest in four or five weeks? It was quickly confirmed that the donation date would probably be on January 8, less than a month away.

I was fortunate to have a supportive work environment and some flexibility in my work schedule. I traveled to a specialized clinic two hours from my home for a comprehensive physical, which included an EKG (electrical study of the heart), x-rays, complete blood work (eight vials!) and a general well-being check from the staff. I viewed the experience as an excellent baseline health data for my life and appreciated the experience. I took interest in my own health and enjoyed learning details about the functioning of body systems. I was also fortunate that the Be The Match Foundation (and my recipient's insurance) funded all the costs of these tests including mileage to the facility and all associated costs.

On December 11, I was informed the stem cell harvest would indeed take place on January 8. I coordinated with the Be the Match Foundation for appropriate travel to the harvesting location, about five hours from my home.

As a blood-products donor, I was familiar and comfortable with the process. Any discomfort was tolerable when I considered the extraordinary implications. For five days before the donation, I was given a drug called Neupogen, used to stimulate the bone marrow production process. It had to be injected by a nurse, and I had to be monitored for fifteen minutes after the shot, to ensure there was no allergic reaction, the most common side effect.

At this point, the thought of a potential allergic reaction was one of the only times during the process that I had any pause for thought.

The list of side effects for the drug was fairly comprehensive, as is with any medication one takes; however because of the somewhat limited clinical use and narrow therapeutic index, I was a bit worried about the side effects. They ranged from anaphylaxis (an allergic reaction that can stop you from breathing and be fatal) to a spleen rupture, which they were so kind as to indicate was also sometimes fatal.

I was given paperwork to sign indicating that I agreed to the voluntary procedure, and as with any surgery or procedure, it had inherent risks, up to and including death. I was asked to fill out my advanced directive and religious preferences. Again, a very, very small chance of anything bad happening, but certainly it gave me something to consider and discuss with my family.

The procedure was done using a process called apheresis. Essentially, instead of drilling a large bore needle into my hip bone and extracting the bone marrow itself, the Neupogen drug caused a massive increase of free-formed bone marrow in my blood. The blood was taken out of my vein through a large, but still standard, needle in my right arm. It then went into a machine that separated the bone marrow from my blood and plasma and returned both to me, along with saline and calcium, to reduce the tingling effects of the anticoagulant. I slept through half of the donation and watched TV the other half.

I saw a bag of yellow substance get whisked away and wondered what happened thereafter. Bone marrow has a forty-eight-hour shelf life. I learned it was overnighted, further tested, and administered within twenty-four hours. My eight hours of harvest time netted 12 million stem cells, an excess over the need, allowing HCI to save four million stem cells for any future need the recipient might have. This news was excellent, because if for some reason the patient ever relapsed, he would be able to have a transplant immediately, instead of having to coordinate with me and use my cells again. In essence, he still has some of me in the bank. I also consented for a small portion of the stem cells to be used for genetic research, as I am happy to oblige and further medical science in any way that I can. At the time, however, I did not know where the stem cells went or who received them. It was completely anonymous.

I felt tired for a few days as my body replaced the shortfall of stem cells. I was back to work in two days and felt normal within a week.

Good Attention to the Donor

The process was well organized. It didn't cost me anything. All costs, including lost wages, were covered by the recipient's insurance. The registry was committed to safeguarding and supporting my health during the process and addressing any related health needs for two years thereafter. Part of the process was regular phone reviews afterwards, to make sure that I was back to good health.

My contact person was attentive and friendly. Nothing was impersonal about the registry process. In fact, the main aspect I appreciated the most wasn't necessarily the financial reimbursement, but the ease in which the foundation organized everything for me. I was busy working, and as much as I wanted to help, I couldn't take a whole lot of time for planning. The registry was able to tell me what/when/where and I was quite thankful for that.

The needed disclosures of the process and all medications, and a request for legal health and life documents to be in order, for liability purposes and practical disclosure, did give me a moment's pause for thought; another level of awareness that there is a risk to everything. I can understand how some people might find the details daunting and perhaps change their mind.

I was confident in my good health at my young age. I understood that my health could change and I could have a need in the future. We need to do what we can. This experience gave me some perspective of change that can happen.

This Is It—The Real Deal
The Transplant

Fred's E-mail Communications

If you don't give people information,
they'll make up something to fill the void.
- Carla Odell

A friend is someone who knows the song of your soul
and sings it back to you when you've forgotten the words.
- Unknown

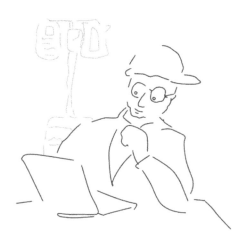

Transplant: Day 0 to Day 100

NOTE: Prior to the stem cell transplant, everyone's treatment differs, based on the patient's diagnosis, symptoms, reaction to chemo, etc. Once the stem cell process starts (Day 0), everyone has the same Day 0 to Day 100 general plan.

We used e-mail to communicate with family and friends. In this section we are using "Fred Updates" to highlight key events as well as to illustrate how we communicated to family and friends.

We often started our e-mails with the following:

THANKS again for all of your prayers and good wishes. We know they are working because everything is progressing.

The e-mails always ended with this:

GAME ON!

CHARDI KALA – Sikh sentiment: high and soaring spirits; positive and optimistic attitude to life and the future

SUCCESS = Physical Condition, Mental and Spiritual Preparation, Steadfast Optimism

Final Preparation for the Stem Cell Transplant

Fred Update–Stem Cell Transplant Schedule

Here's our planned schedule:

January 3 - check into HCI to start pre-transplant chemo to eliminate all of my bone marrow.

January 9 - my new birthdate. I will receive the donor's stem cells by a transfusion of stem cells over two hours.

After the January 3rd round of chemo I will become incapable of producing new blood cells. In fourteen to twenty-one days after the transplant my body will accept the donor stem cells and start producing new blood cells. We will know the donor stem cells are working when my blood tests start showing positive results.

In four to six weeks, once my immune systems hits a minimum level (ANC = 500), I will be discharged from the hospital.

Through Day 100 - After the donor's stem cells start working, there is a new risk of GVHD (Graft-Versus-Host Disease), in which the new, transplanted cells regard the recipient's body as foreign. When this happens, the newly transplanted cells attack the recipient's body. GVHD can be mild, moderate, severe, and even life threatening. (www.medlineplus.com)

The staff has stressed that the first month will be difficult because of the combination of intense chemo and a war going on inside my body as the donor stem cells invade my system. They have emphasized that I need to concentrate on three simple tasks: eating, drinking, and exercising.

In summary we are READY and we are OPTIMISTIC. We are looking forward to getting this health issue behind us.

BTW, we skied on New Year's Day just prior to my being admitted as an inpatient for the transplant. The Utah-based snow angels blessed us with more than seven feet of snow, allowing us to enjoy good skiing before my season was put on hold. We skied seven days in the past two weeks. YES!! My goal is to be back on the ski slopes in March, sixty days after the transplant!

E-mail from Ohtani-san, a good friend from Japan.

Roth san:

A Happy New Year.

It is our custom to pay our first visit of the year to temples or shrines during the first three days of the new year.

Today, I went to Narita-san Temple with my wife, which is located near Narita International Airport. This temple is one of the most famous temples in Japan. Visiting people like to buy small pieces of holy wood from the temple and write their New Year's wishes, such as safety of family, healthy body, happy marriage, business success, etc., on the wood. The temple priest burns this holy wood in front of Buddhist statues to grant wishes and requests.

Today we wrote "the healthy body of my wife and me, the safety of my son's family, and the heart's desire of my daughter, who wishes to have a baby" on the three pieces of holy wood. On the fourth holy wood, we wrote "the healthy body of Fred Roth-san."

We hope our wishes will reach the God's heart.

Keep in touch.

Katsumi Ohtani

Fred Update—Countdown to Day 0

The big day is tomorrow! This morning the doctors gave their GO to proceed, so no roadblocks prevent us from moving to Day 0!

My BMT doctor's concluding comment at today's meeting – "you are ready!"

He believed the delays worked in my favor, in that I was able to build up my strength and go into the process in good condition. All systems are now GO for my new birth on January 9.

A lot of the staff members came in to wish me the best for tomorrow.

I finished seven days on intense chemo to destroy all of my bone marrow. I made it through with minimal problems, except for one bad overnight stretch reacting to the chemo.

The stem-cell harvesting has already been completed by the donor and is now en route overnight to the hospital. THANK YOU, Donor #12!

Glad we're finally moving to Day 0 after six months of waiting!

GAME ON. YES!!

Fred's Lessons Learned

- Count down to transplant day—the most important day of your NEXT life.
- Stay positive: You are approaching your first day of recovery. We skied the day prior to being admitted for the transplant. We were enjoying every day and anticipating a good life ahead.
- Prepare for the transplant
  - » Mentally: Be optimistic. You need this transplant to survive, so do anything in your power to make it work. Ask yourself, "What do I have to do, and how do I have to prepare for success?"
  - » Physically: Get in shape, Exercise like your life depends on it, because it does.
- I needed to be in good condition with my body systems strong and with some extra weight through healthy nutrition.

Stem Cell Transplant—Day 0 to Day 36

Fred Update—Day 0

Yes, we finally made it to Day 0!

The doctors started the process using comments about the stem-cell collection that included "outstanding" and "excellent," which definitely made us feel optimistic.

A good stem-cell collection contains six million cells. My donor was very generous with 12 million stem cells. The doctors decided to give me eight million and freeze four million in case I needed it later.

This was my twelfth potential donor; he/she said yes on 12/12/12 and gave me 12 million stem cells. Number twelve is truly my lucky number.

We celebrated this occasion as the beginning. Kathy and friends decorated the room. We had music.

The process started at 1:30 p.m. MST and took two hours. I received the stem cells through an IV from a bag of the donor's red blood. The staff closely monitored my blood pressure and temperature to make sure I was not having an immediate negative reaction.

All the staff members sang Happy Birthday as we started the transfer. It's an appropriate song, because going forward they no longer care about my real birthday; everything is measured and tracked from Day 0.

The next challenge is for my body to accept the donor's cells during the next fourteen to twenty-one days. It's a matter of waiting, reviewing daily blood tests, and monitoring the changes.

We were forewarned that the next three weeks could get very nasty, with major fatigue and other issues. We just need to dig in until I am over the hump and start to recover.

The doctors all agree I am ready to move forward. YES!

Fred Update - Day 1

Just a short note to let you know we had a good Day 1. No problems. Good energy and appetite.

Doctors congratulated me on a great Day 1 but to expect lesser days ahead, so we are warned and ready.

Fred Update - Day 5

Day 5, and I'm still feeling good. Good appetite and mild fatigue. The medical staff keeps warning me that I will soon go over a "cliff," but so far I don't see or feel any cliff. I am walking each day in the BMT confined hallways. I cannot leave the immediate BMT area, so my walking path is limited. Thanks to my Fitbit activity tracker, I know my distance traveled! I am also Fitbit friends with several nurses.

Per our friend Joel's excellent advice, I am taking it one day at a time, and each day so far has been good.

Fred Update - Day 7

Wow! One week, and I'm still doing well.

I worked very hard to strengthen my body, heart, and lungs prior to the transplant.

Doctors are enthusiastic, so we remain optimistic. The next key dates will be between Day 14 and Day 28, when there should be evidence that Fred 2.0 is taking over with improved blood counts. Stay tuned!

Karl, my brother-in-law, started calling me Fred 2.0 after I received the donor's stem cells. The name caught on, so the new Fred is Fred 2.0.

Fred Update - Day 10

Day 10, and I am still doing well. I am walking several miles daily in tight confines. I need to watch my timing not to interfere with hallway traffic. The doctors ask how I'm feeling, and I respond with my mileage totals. They are satisfied with my answer.

My immune system is now completely shut down and Fred-1 is gone. Goodbye, Fred-1. You were very good to me.

Now we wait as Fred 2.0 starts protecting me at some point in the next one to two weeks. We will know he is with me when the blood tests show improvement.

A side effect of the chemo and transplant is mouth and throat sores (mucositis). They started yesterday, and it became difficult to eat and talk. Unfortunately the sores will remain until my immune system returns in one to two weeks, so I will be on a liquid diet and I will not be talking much for the next week or so.

Fred Update – Day 11

Sonia knows best. I have been trying to tough it out with the mucositis, but Nurse Sonia convinced me that I should try a suction system for mucus and saliva. It helped some. I also had the option of a pain pump. I reduced my walking schedule, as I need to take a few catnaps with this pain management.

Fred Update - Day 12

Good news! Fred-1 shut down on Day 10, and Fred 2.0 started kicking in. Mouth sores are still troublesome. Ugh!

Today's blood tests showed a very small blood count recovery, but any improvement is good news.

Fred Update - Day 15

Luckily Fred 2.0 is jumping in to help me. Today my ANCs made a big jump to 900. YES! This is very good news.

The bad news this week is that since I hit bottom, a large number of mouth and throat sores developed, because I have no immune system to slow them down. For the past week I could not eat or talk. The primary problem is the sores caused my throat to swell and there was minimal passage into my throat. Even pain medicine did not allow me to eat, because of the swelling.

Finally after five days with zero food and liquid, today I am able to drink two energy drinks to give me about 1,000 calories. I am on a fluid IV to make sure I get enough liquids, but the hospital prefers not use food IV, because of side effects. If the doctors think you are strong enough, they recommend simply not eating until the swelling decreases, instead of using food IV.

Fred Update - Day 18

Everything is now improving, and we're back on track. The mouth and throat sores are much better. It was a brutal week, but I can now eat and talk with limitations. I am still walking three miles daily.

My blood counts continue to improve. My ANCs have been over 2,000 for three days, which is fantastic. I have not needed any blood infusions recently, because Fred 2.0 is pumping out a lot of new blood. YES!

Doctors are now talking about letting me head home soon. FANTASTIC!

We had Stanley Steamer clean our condo carpets and furniture yesterday, a requirement before I can return home.

Life is good again!

Fred Update - Day 19 – HOME!

YES! Coming home in nineteen days is a fantastic gift!

This morning during the doctor rounds, doctors said to start packing, because there was no reason to stay any longer. Kathy and I are doing a lot of hugging and crying today. We are both in tears as we write this note.

We remain convinced what got us here today was physical conditioning and my fighter's mindset, steadfast optimism, and the world-class HCI facility.

We still have a very long and unknown road ahead of us, but we have achieved a major, major, major objective today.

It's been a difficult seven-month journey that included eighty-two days as an inpatient, twenty-five days of chemo, and significant other challenges, including finding a committed donor.

A special thanks to Donor #12. We hope we have the opportunity to thank you in person.

Fred Update - Day 35 – Speed Bumps: Back as Inpatient

I was home for a week but then needed to return to the hospital with problems.

I was admitted back as an inpatient for ten days. I encountered a stomach infection, lower esophagus inflammation, and pancreatitis. All issues are now resolved, so we have no concerns going forward. They do not know the cause of the pancreatitis. I just know it was very painful.

I hope to go home tomorrow. I could have gone home today, but yesterday I did not consume enough liquids or calories. I have to demonstrate that I can eat 1,500 calories and drink two liters of fluid. I could not, yesterday, so I have another day as an inpatient. Today my appetite is back. I ate and drank my requirement so we fully expect to head home tomorrow, Valentine's Day.

Fred Update - Day 36 – Home Again

Valentine's Day, and I am back home again. The best Valentine's gift ever!

Fred's Lessons Learned

- The Big Day, Fred 2.0's birth! We celebrate the first day of my recovery. Celebrate! Don't despair—welcome those new stem cells into your body. Feel them going through you. The start of the new Fred 2.0.
- After the transplant my primary focus was exercising, eating, and drinking. I concentrated on getting this situation behind us.
- Exercised—walked, walked, walked, and used the stationary bike in my hospital room.
- I made sure the doctors saw me exercising—walking (almost running) in the hallways and pedaling on the exercise bike. They knew they had a motivated patient.
- We watched the numbers, tracked the blood counts and kept a daily diary.
- The ANCs tanked to zero and then slowly crept back to 500. With no white blood cells, the risk of bad things increased.
- ANC: Absolute Neutrophil Count, the number of white blood cells (WBCs) that are neutrophils. Neutrophils are key components in the system of defense against infection. An absence or scarcity of neutrophils (neutropenia) makes a person vulnerable to infection. After chemo or a blood or marrow transplant, the ANC is usually depressed and then slowly rises, reflecting the fact that the bone marrow is recovering and new blood cells are beginning to grow and mature. (www.medicinenet.com)
- It was very concerning when white blood cells and ANCs did not start generating. We rejoiced when the ANCs finally moved above zero and slowly started marching toward 500.

"ANCs were just clunking along" was a quote from one of our favorite doctors.

- My appetite disappeared when the ANCs tanked until they were back over 500.
- I sometimes felt fatigued as my body started working hard to integrate with the new stem cells. I stayed out of bed no matter how bad I felt. I kept exercising to help get my new stem cells circulating.
- Mask: Walking the halls with a hospital mask was difficult. Although it kept the germs out, it kept the carbon dioxide from my breath in. After about ten minutes with the ubiquitous paper masks, I needed to go into my room just to breathe. Patient and friend John, a long distance runner, found RESPRO Mask, a high-tech mask manufactured in Britain. It's a bit pricey but much better than the hospital paper masks. He runs long distance with this mask. Visit www.johnnyrunner.com for more information and order instructions.

- The dreaded **mucositis**
  » Mucositis: Inflammation of the mucous membranes lining the digestive tract from the mouth to the anus. www.medicinenet.com
  » Mucositis is a common side effect of chemo. Mucositis affects the rapidly dividing mucosal cells that line the mouth, throat, stomach, and intestines, which normally have a short lifespan. If a therapy destroys these cells, they may not be replaced right away, in which case mucositis results. A person with mucositis may have raw sores (ulcers) in the mouth, throat and beyond. It can feel like he or she has sunburn in the throat. www.medicinenet.com
  » Relate this unpleasant period to simply having the flu for two weeks, feeling lousy and not being able to eat.
  » When I could not eat because of mouth sores, I survived for two weeks on yogurt and healthy smoothies.

- » Just get through it. There is little you can do except manage the pain and wait it out.
- I had ups and downs. Every day was a new one. I tried not to get depressed. Feeling tired and ill is part of the recovery journey. It was a short-term problem in a long-term solution.
- The first one hundred days were critical. Per my sister-in-law's recommendation, I used percentages instead of days, 10% of the way to one hundred days, 25% of the way to one hundred days, etc.
- I sent frequent e-mail updates to family and friends. Every day was an important one.
- **SUMMARY:** Be kind to yourself and rest when needed, but be truthful. It's easy just to lie in bed and do nothing. In your heart, you know you can do something productive. Tie up the sneakers, order room service for fuel and nutrition, and ring for more water. Make good things happen.

STRIVING TO DAY 100–Birth of Fred 2.0

Fred Update - Day 50

Day 50, 50% of the way to my critical one-hundred-day mark! Status update–doing well:

- **Weight**–I lost twenty-five pounds during the transplant process. I intentionally went into the hospital for the transplant ten pounds over my normal weight, hence a net loss of only fifteen pounds. I am slowly getting my appetite back and starting to recover some of the weight lost.
- **Physical Condition**–I lost a lot of muscle tone and am now trying to get it back.
- **Skiing**–I asked one of my doctors if I could ski soon. She said OK once I felt physically able. I was careful who I asked permission for skiing. I asked only the doctor that I knew was a gung-ho skier to improve my chances of getting permission!

Fred Update - Days 60–62—SKIING!

A very important goal we established before the transplant was to be back on the ski slopes in two months. We achieved our objective on Days 60 to 62, exactly two months!

I worked very hard to get my muscle strength back again. I walked for miles. I did stairs two and three times a day. My legs felt great all three days of easy skiing, so I was back in good shape.

Utah skiing in March can be excellent and the Utah Weather Angels came through for us this week. There was good snow, warm temperatures, deep blue sky, and bright sun. We skied at Deer Valley with our good friends Jerry and Claudia. Priceless!

Fred Update - Day 75

Day 75, 75% of the way to Day 100! We are taking it one day at a time. Transplant day (Day 0) seemed years away from Day 100. Suddenly it is almost here.

A nurse asked if we had plans for our 100-day celebration. We had not thought about it. Kathy and I immediately decided on a trip to Moab in Southern Utah to hike in the national parks.

Now I had a new goal to achieve, to be ready to hike to Delicate Arch in Arches National Park on Day 100 to celebrate.

We discussed with our doctor the topic of immunizations and vaccinations. All of the vaccinations I received since childhood are gone. Starting at one year we will begin vaccinations, and it will take six months to complete the process. We will have the same vaccination schedule for shots as a one-year-old baby.

I am still taking strong immune suppressants to reduce the risk of organ rejection. We will start reducing these on Day 100 and gradually reduce them for the next six months. During this timeframe there is an increased risk of organ problems as a result of rejection of the new stem cells, so I will be closely monitored.

Fred Update - Day 85

The critical Day 100 mark is rapidly approaching—85% of the way there!

I had a full day of "Day 100" tests, including dental, lungs, chest x-ray, heart-strength tests, blood tests, and a bone-marrow biopsy. Our big meeting with our BMT doctor will be next week when we will discuss test results and determine a plan for moving forward.

Fred Update - Day 86

Our BMT doctor called this morning. He just received my bone-marrow biopsy results and did not want to wait until our Wednesday meeting to give us the good news.

He started the conversation using "splendid" and "perfect." He, too, was excited about the outcome after his hard work and that of the staff. No sign of any leukemia. I am now officially in remission!

Fred Update - Day 90

Today is Day 90, and we had our "Day 100" doctor meeting.

Thankfully all test results are very positive. The most significant was the bone-marrow biopsy results: no sign of any leukemia, officially in remission. My blood is now 96% Fred 2.0, a strong count for this stage.

The doctors are excited about our results and share the excitement that they progress in the work against this disease.

We now know the donor is male. My bone marrow biopsy showed that I still have XY chromosomes. If it had been a female donor, I would now have XX chromosomes.

Moving Forward/More Work Ahead

The next phase is to reduce my medications over the next six months. The challenge is for organ acceptance of the new blood system. The goal is to have a healthy system operating naturally without chemical intervention. The focus for the next six months will be rebuilding my immunization. I currently have the immune system of a 90-day-old baby. Infections continue to be a risk.

Fred Update - Day 98

To celebrate our 100 Day milestone we took six dozen bagels to the BMT staff.

We have three groups that we are indebted to for their fine work, Pre-BMT, BMT, and outpatient clinic. We were at the hospital with the bagels at 6:30 a.m. to catch the night shift and arriving day shift. Several nurses teared up during our celebration. I can now accept hugs (!), and I started collecting on my hug IOUs today from the nurses.

Fred Update - Day 100!

Day 100 was a distant target on Day 0, and now it's here with excellent results.

To celebrate this good fortune, we spent five days hiking at the Arches and Canyonlands National Parks in Southern Utah.

Canyonlands is the Utah version of the Grand Canyon, 2,000 feet above the Colorado River.

We looked forward to our hike to Delicate Arch, a dazzling formation that is the state symbol. It's an interesting hike through rock formations to a dramatic vista. The gift of the trip was thirty minutes of solitude at the arch before anyone else arrived, a quiet moment to appreciate.

The next challenge is the gradual withdrawal of supportive medications over the next six months. Meanwhile, my immune system (now only 100 days old) needs to rebuild. There is still a bumpy road ahead but we continue to be very optimistic.

Thanks again for all of your outstanding support. Every day someone reached out and offered love and encouragement. That extra touch always reminded us that we were not alone. We are ever grateful. Know we are here for you.

I see a life's mission developing. I never thought I would be good at something like this but I'm clearly headed toward helping other cancer patients. I am now coaching several new patients and getting a lot of satisfaction from it. It is a sobering experience, as some are struggling with their recovery. My assistance is appreciated by the patients, families, doctors, and nurses.

Fred's Lessons Learned

- I needed to focus on simply surviving the first critical one hundred days.
- Side effects: fatigue, no appetite, no taste buds, infections.
- Battle of Fred 1.0 versus Fred 2.0: This battle took a lot of energy. It required real fuel. It required helpful fuel. Comfort foods were sometimes in order. Sugar provides intense calories, but no nutrients, a negative that needs to be washed out but presents calories. Be mindful that you are asking your body to do more work. Your mind thinks that these comfort foods will take you to a happy place.
- I tried to stay positive / challenged when the bad things happened.
- I strived to add weight by eating healthy foods.
- We all have delicate skin after the transplant. Ivory soap helped reduce the skin irritation. According to the Ivory soap website, "This isn't your grandmother's soap. This is your great-great-grandmother's soap! For 130 years, we've brought simple, effective cleaning products to families everywhere. If it's good enough for Nana, it's good enough for you!"
- Create high-quality time. Every day you are alive is a great day. Enjoy the sunrises and sunsets.
- "Fred sitters" - You need a support system after you are discharged and at home. You cannot be left alone during the first 100 days. You need to be within thirty minutes of the hospital.
- We set goals with specific dates:

» Skied on Days 60, 61, 62. Priceless! Important mental victory to be back on the slopes.

» Day 100, celebrated! We climbed to Delicate Arch in Arches National Park, thirty minutes alone at this beautiful sight, a quiet, peaceful celebration.

» I wanted to make those Fred 2.0 stem cells appreciate an active body.

Donor Perspectives After The Transplant

Written by Chris, our donor

We need to do what we can.
- Chris

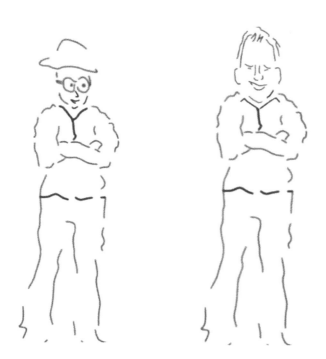

Contact with the recipient

After my involvement I would periodically receive filtered communications that the recipient appeared to have a good response and was regaining strength. After one year I received a request for contacting the recipient, one that I could accept or decline.

Many people are not interested in hearing anything about their recipient. Often, through no fault of the donor, the recipient doesn't make it. This result can be an emotionally devastating thing for donors, as they can feel survivor's guilt and wonder if they did something wrong. Many donors wish to donate and then just assume it is in someone else's capable hands and out of theirs. I was curious about the other side of the process and knew that there was a very real possibility that the person I donated to would not survive. To me, the not knowing would have been much more agonizing than knowing one way or another.

Fred and his wife offered to come to thank me in person, meeting my family and me over an evening's dinner at a hotel in my home city (March 1, one year and two months post-transplant). It was an emotional experience to see a healthy-looking man in good spirits and know that I played an important part in his current existence.

Visit to Huntsman Cancer Institute

I received Fred's family-and-friends general updates after we met on March 1. I was very curious about the other side of the process.

I contacted Fred to see if I could visit HCI. I flew to Salt Lake City to tour the extraordinary facility and spent twelve hours over two days meeting staff with Kathy and Fred. Fred and the donor coordinators organized a schedule to meet more than fifty staff members who found time to connect as well as attend an informal reception in the BMT conference room.

The tone for the visit was set by our first contact, a senior nurse who said, "You will be told over and over that you are wonderful and awesome and you are. Just take it all in and say thank you."

Many staff members used my name before I was introduced, as they recognized me from the posted notices throughout the hospital. Every person was warm, enthusiastic, and generous with their hugs. I was a celebrity for the two days. As one nurse explained, "You don't know how many lives you touched with your generosity."

As we prepared to leave, a young nurse rode the elevator with us. She said she had been at the hospital for only two months but she knew who we were and our story. "You are a VIP!"

I find this process fascinating. My cells can power another body and renew life. I initially viewed this act as a good deed but now I have the sense that it is miraculous technology still in its developing stages.

I was amazed at the entire process of the donation and care for the recipient of my bone marrow. I had a general idea of the process but didn't realize it took only a few hours to inject the bone marrow into Fred's body, literally a reverse of the procedure I did. I also didn't realize the staggering scope of the operation required in order to ensure a patient's survival. Every member is of *vital* importance, down to the person cleaning the room. Sanitation and sterilization can easily make the difference between life and death. Nurses, assistants, dietitians, physical therapists, nutritionists, and administrative staff; the list of contributors goes on. Each contribution is as important as the other and in no politically correct terms, but in actual reality terms.

The choreography of coordinating each step of the way was nothing short of remarkable. It is very easy to get complacent in our jobs but I don't think anyone I met would even consider their work to be a job. It's just what they do and what they love. I don't think you can work in that kind of industry without some kind of passion for it, as burn-out rates for the medical facility are staggering. Some of the nurses there had been there more than twenty years. For a cancer facility, the longevity of the staff is unbelievable.

I now look for opportunities to use my donor experience to spread the word to "Be the Match." I have a better understanding of the importance of a bank of young, healthy donors, particularly women and ethnic donors. I have discussions about the donor process when the opportunities arise, with business colleagues who inquired about my travel plans and conversations with my plane seatmate en route to Salt Lake City. I am sure that my gift bag of HCI souvenirs given to me will provide impetus for conversations at home. Currently I have the HCI water bottle on my desk, and I'll make a poignant effort to take it to any meetings I go to.

I also just reconfirmed my recommitment to the registry. I'm good to go as an anonymous donor again. I'm happy to help for as long as I can, as the registry generally doesn't take anonymous donations past forty-five years of age. I hope the next generation is ready to take up the mantle.

Kathy's comments: If "It takes a village to raise a child," it takes a village to support a donor.

Having met Chris and his family, I understood the supporting role that others play in the donor process. Chris's father was his role model. His father had donated blood since his twenties. Chris often accompanied his dad for this task and began donating when he was of age. In their family it's what men do. He expanded his donation abilities as needed.

Chris's employer was generous in providing time and flexibility. Undoubtedly his work colleagues assisted in covering for him during his absence.

One can imagine other tasks that might be needed: child care, driving, etc.

Encourage the young people in your life to Be the Match. Let them know that you proudly support their commitment and are there to assist them in this undertaking.

Replies to Fred's Update E-mail Regarding Chris's visit to HCI

From family and friends:

- Thanks, Chris, for your selfless act! You were the answer to many prayers!
- It does sound like an amazing weekend. I think of all the donors you went through to get to Chris, how frustrating it was at the time, but how it was part of God's plan. What a great example for me of God's sovereignty. Thanks for sharing.
- Great e-mail! We were thinking about you the whole weekend. So glad you saw so many special people at HCI. Surely a rewarding experience for the staff to be part of such a wonderful story.
- I find it very special that you were able to connect with him at this level, take him to the facility that allowed the doctors to make the process play out, and then for Chris to meet and touch the very people who assisted in saving your life.
- What a beautiful heartwarming story. Chris is included in our daily prayers, for his kindness, greatness, and selfless donation for saving Fred's life. People like him make this world a great place. May he always be blessed with good health and happiness.
- Greetings from Shanghai. Your news brought tears to my eyes. What a great story. Spreading this story brings more to the infinite benefits that Chris provided with his selfless act and your response to it by sharing hope to so many who are in desperate need. XO Thanks for keeping in touch.
- I can only imagine how emotional it must have been for you and Kathy, and how appropriate that it was Easter/Passover weekend. Faith, renewed life, new beginnings—perfect. I can't help but think of all the hope you and Chris must have given those new patients.

- This is such an amazing story of how you and Chris have had an impact on the lives of so many people at HCI, Fred. That ripple effect is being felt in a positive way in so many ways. Isn't life so amazing?
- Three superstars together in one place! What a life-altering event for you and Kathy. How often does a life-threatening event turn into a blessing? Your life has changed in so many wonderful ways. Continues to be a great story.
- What an incredible bond you and Chris share! You are truly blessed in many ways. Thank you for sharing.
- Caring and sharing–that's what life is all about, right? Sounds like a wonderful time with Chris. You are really an inspiration to us all. I love hearing from you.
- Awesome, awesome, awesome! You are an inspiration to soooooooooooooo many! Well deserved! Awesome you and Chris are now friends! New patient orientation–those you meet don't know what a blessing that is! You're the best!
- It is often your uplifting e-mails that make my day. It sure did today
- Your story carries on well outside of SLC as I tell it to many people I come across as a great example of what a positive attitude can do.

From HCI Management and Administration

- Thanks for sharing the pictures. What a great experience for everyone involved. It was an honor to meet Chris.
- It was exciting for the staff to meet Chris as a real person and not a faceless, nameless donor with an assigned number. They got to witness his interaction with you and Kathy. The visit also piqued the staff's interest about volunteering to be a donor. In addition, it buoyed their spirits knowing that we have many success stories such as yours. Thank you for all you do for HCI, the patients, and staff.

- What a great story. I'm going to include your pictures and a brief description of your meeting in my weekly HCI blog. Thanks for being such a great advocate for the staff and future patients. We are blessed that you connected with Chris's stem cells and have continued to have a relationship with HCI.
- I am so glad it all went so well for you and Chris to come to HCI. It has been an honor to have been part of your treatment through transplant. Your case of trying to find a donor will always be close to my heart and a memorable experience.
- It was nice of you to track me down so I would get the opportunity to meet Chris. I know how much of an incredible experience this has been for you, and I'm glad you were able to meet your donor. I want to be a donor!

Optimism About Life And The Future!

I am reclaiming my strength.
- Affirmation

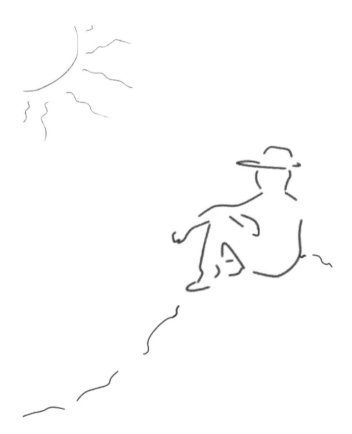

Striving for that first Birthday

- Be alert, be aware, and be conservative, but not too conservative.
- Exercise–even when you don't want to.
- Eat healthy–nourishment for the "new" you.
- Food you used to like, you won't like for weeks or months. Luckily those good tastes will return.
- Stay in contact with your friends and fellow patients. Fred's support team: Four amigos who all walked the hallways together.
- Infections, GVHD: Keep listening to your doctor's advice and keep taking your meds.
- If something looks or feels different, see your medical team. Don't be macho. Get that TLC from your medical team.
- Stay positive–you will get over these short-term bumps.
- Enjoy each day–you are alive!
- Mentor others who are just starting their journey. You can coach them on the road they are about to travel. You are now the expert. Patients will appreciate your guidance.

Tips for Avoiding Conflict (Source: Be The Match Registry)

- When something rubs you the wrong way, think about the person's intent and let it go.
- Ask for clarification to avoid misunderstanding.
- Tell people how you feel–be honest.
- Discuss how things could be done differently.
- Spend time with those who help you stay positive.
- Reduce stress by taking good care of yourself.

Moving From Surviving To Living (Source: Be The Match Registry)

- What do you want your life to be like going forward?
- There is life after a transplant!
- Recover a sense of control over your life.
- Never have a bad day.
- Love stronger, care more, play harder.
- Am I living the life I want to live?
- How have my priorities changed?

Cancer is so limited (from a sign in each HCI patient room)

- It cannot cripple LOVE
- It cannot shatter HOPE
- It cannot corrode FAITH
- It cannot destroy PEOPLE
- It cannot kill FRIENDSHIP
- It cannot suppress MEMORIES
- It cannot silence COURAGE
- It cannot invade the SOUL
- It cannot steal eternal LIFE
- It cannot conquer the SPIRIT

More about the masks

SPORTSTA MASK (www.johnnyrunner.com)
- I needed to wear a mask in public for the first one hundred days to keep from breathing bad things.
- Buy a high-tech mask. You will look cool, and it's much more comfortable. SPORTSTA MASK (www.johnnyrunner.com).
- I still wear a mask on planes. I don't have to, but it keeps cold and flu germs way. I explain to my seatmates why I wear it, and they always reply that they often get sick after long flights and

they should wear one. It has kept me from picking up bugs on flights, and it often generates interesting discussions.
- To start the conversation with "About the mask, I want to assure you that I do not have anything that's contagious. Rather I am worried about all of you and picking up a cold. I am happy to say I am recovering from an immunity issue."

Long term objectives—looking FORWARD!

- Reflect on your journey. Celebrate having achieved a miracle.
- I've been given a second life. What do I want to do with it?
- **Mentor.** Share your story. We are thankful for what HCI provided.
- **Help others in need, the giving side of Chardi Kala.** Pay it forward. I am paying back my mentor, Bruce, who was there for me in my darkest days. Others can benefit from your experience.
- Suggest that others donate through the National Registry. They can share their good health.
- Support systems: employer, family, friends. It takes many to make it happen. They think you're worth it.
- Document your annual physical exams.
- Keep the exercise routines going. Continue with an ongoing healthy lifestyle.
- Continue eating healthy foods.
- Continue closely watching your health, your weight, blood pressure, cholesterol levels, and any change in your condition. Continue taking recommended medications.
- Stay connected with family and friends. Reunions now have a much greater meaning and importance! Make more effort to stay connected.

Six-Month, One-Year AND BEYOND Celebrations

- You are still ALIVE!
- CELEBRATE every milestone!

- Share the celebrations with family and friends—they want to celebrate with you.
- You now have two birthdays. Celebrate both!
- Receiving the "one-year old" birthday cards, cherished baby cards!
- Receiving the one-year vaccinations—same schedule as one-year-old babies!
- Your chances of survival have now dramatically improved.
- You are living proof that the effort was worth it.
- Today is a gift. That's why it's called the present.
- Every day is a GREAT DAY!
- CELEBRATE LIFE!

Our Chardi Kala friends, the Gills, brought forward the analogy of climbing a mountain. You see the peak and know that is your destination. There is no IMAX version for this experience. You know it will be difficult, requiring extraordinary effort and likely pain. You commit. You plan your strategy. You enlist resources. You begin the journey. Every day you work toward the peak. Sometimes bad weather blows in and you hunker down. You strategically rest. You move forward at every opportunity.

Climb your mountain!

We cheer you on!

Good science, good care, good blessings, good luck - and good effort on your part!

Second Transplant

Oh, Boo!
(and many other statements of like sentiment)
- Fred

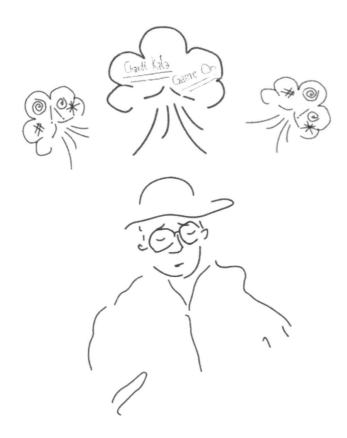

The saga continues: leukemia relapse and second stem cell transplant.

It was July, three years after my Leukemia diagnosis and 2.5 years since receiving Chris's stem cells.

Life was back to normal, and I was enjoying every single day. Events that used to irritate me no longer mattered. My priorities were very different and I had a different view of the world. I was traveling for business and pleasure. I was mentoring cancer patients and found this work greatly gratifying. Life was very, very good.

Every six weeks I had a clinic appointment with blood tests to confirm everything was normal. In mid-July I had a routine clinic appointment and I was confident there were no issues. My doctor for the appointment was new, and we had never met. After the blood tests were completed he asked how I was feeling. I replied I was doing excellently and felt great. He asked me again how I felt, and I replied with the same answer.

I could tell by the look on his face that he was not agreeing with my reply. I firmly asked why he appeared concerned. He said one of my blood counts was off. Being a "numbers guy," I immediately asked which blood count and what was the specific count. My white blood cells had tanked and my ANCs were suddenly less than 500. What? How can that be?

I must have turned ashen in color, because the nurse asked if I was OK and whether I wanted to sit down. I was in shock. Not again. Those tests could not be accurate. Perhaps my tests were mixed up with someone else's.

The head doctor entered the room and said it was clear I had relapsed. As before, my only solution was a stem cell transplant.

I was scared once again. I was very fortunate to have fully recovered from my first transplant. Can I make it two miracles? I was fearful that the odds were greatly diminished for someone to go through a second transplant at sixty-five years of age.

Two days later I was admitted back as an inpatient to start the induction chemo followed by a stem cell transplant in mid-September. Chris, our fantastic donor, once again agreed to provide his stem cells.

The BMT staff members took my relapse very hard. They considered me an extension of the nursing staff, because I was often on the floor mentoring patients. Suddenly I was a patient once again.

The results and our story are generally the same as what you have read. I did not have the struggle of the internal viruses and bacteria that live within. Luckily I had minimal mucositis. I did have a double whammy of MRSA and e-coli infections that are common in the outside world. Between the first round of induction chemo and the transplant period I had a 24/7 antibiotic pump for three weeks that I learned to manage. I had ups and downs. I did the same hard work whether I felt like it or not. And now I am back to a full recovery.

Life is good once again, and I am living every day as a new day.

Fred's Lessons Learned

- It can happen again. We are vulnerable.
- I can survive again. We are strong.
- Life can be normal again. We are focused on attitude and effort.
- I am thankful for each day I am given. We live with gratitude.

Appendix

Homefront Notebook

Stress can be the result of death, divorce, or prolonged travel or illness, any event that causes one partner to be "out of the daily loop." Knowing what it takes to keep the household humming helps with stress relief.

Most households generally run on principles of "separation of labor." In the past it might have been gender roles. She did inside housework. He tackled outside yard work. Today, with new tools, the tasks might be shared in different ways, but partners generally claim household jobs by abilities, interests, or tradeoffs. With experience, the "task master" knows the subtleties of each task. The intention is to work together to make life flow efficiently.

And then something happens to disrupt this working system of household harmony. The disruption might be the result of death, divorce, or prolonged illness. Maybe it's just lengthy business travel or out-of-town caregiving. When the information provider is unavailable, a flood of questions begins that revolve around details. What's that account number? Who's the plumber? When is our insurance due? What does our homeowner's insurance cover? How does our health insurance work? Do I know how to interact with the business professionals who are part of our household infrastructure?

Life presents enough disruptive challenges. Building a support system that allows for the sharing of jobs but also provides swapping of responsibilities is about having a family and household process that can be implemented by either partner.

The heart of a process can be a household notebook made up of current statements and contact information grouped in sections.

Examples of our household notebook, a two-inch binder with dividers

When the mail comes in, it takes up space. It suggests action. If you are well organized and work on the principal of "do it now," keep the notebook, a three-hole punch, shredder, and thick black marker nearby. Sort the mail. Punch holes in the most recent statements. Shred the old statements. Block out personal information.

If you have notes that you will likely need later, keep the statement. You do not want to accumulate every monthly statement through the year. In today's world, you can retrieve past statements readily online or from service agents. Having single files for every group of statements never seems to work well, and you end up with cabinets full of paper that eventually get purged as a very big, messy project.

If you live at a fast pace and "let's do it later" fits your flow, have a box or basket nearby with the hole punch and marker in it. Toss the statement there, after you've processed the request for action. Organize the papers later as you watch a movie some low-key evening once a quarter. Have a companion folder for tax information that collects during tax season. Collect receipts and information on other deductible items in the folder as they appear.

As you flip through the notebook, you will have frequent reminders of the business side of your household. Touching these papers helps keep goals in focus and expenditures in view.

Someone mentioned the risk of having the information all in one place. This notebook never leaves the house, although sections might accompany you to meetings with your professionals. It's a bigger risk not to have this information easily accessible.

Here are the notebook categories that reflect the infrastructure of our life.

Residence
- Mortgage information
- Property taxes, check stubs

- Insurance: auto, property, casualty, liability
- Utilities, including cell phone bills
- Car information including a copy of registrations and driver licenses
- Copies of business cards or receipts for workers: plumber, tree service, snow plow service, mowing service, etc.
- Annual expenses list by months (listing/spreadsheet)
- Examples
  - » January: school taxes (estimate $)
  - » February: Car insurance, property insurance (estimate %)
  - » April: AAA renewal
  - » June: annual car inspection with an accompanying sheet that includes hints and tips for getting it done.

Personal Care

- Health insurance statements and due dates
- Life insurance statements and due dates
- Long-term care insurance statements and due dates
- Eye prescriptions
- Medications: Keep photos of your medications on your phone for reference. There are mobile apps that are handy as well, to structure this information. However, your mobile app doesn't help your spouse answer the question of dosage when your phone is left elsewhere.
- Doctor listings: primary care physician, dentist, eye doctor, specialists
- Travel inoculation status (We travel; we're asked)
- Fred keeps a listing of his weight and cholesterol and has done so since age thirty from his annual physical. It was handy when he had his unwanted diagnosis.

Professional Contacts

We keep these together, and we include them in each category. Too many references are better than not enough. These are the folks who help when you need help.

- Investment advisor
- Tax preparer, accountant
- Insurance agent
- Attorney and where the will is located
- Funeral home plans
- Resources you think you might need (cards, flyers, Internet printouts)

Auto

- Copy of Insurance card
- Copy of registration
- Copy of driver's licenses
- Copy of the AAA card, statement, and road service contract
- Insurance statement and payment schedule
- Tires: purchase date, type of tire, air pressure requirements
- Battery: purchase date
- Mechanic contact information and car maintenance history

Finances

- Income information: stubs, contacts
- Bank information: statements, online access (ID, passwords)
- Credit cards: statements, automatic payments, online access (ID, passwords)
- 401(k): statements, online access (ID, passwords)
- Social Security statements (printed from online access)
- Investments: an aggregate page for an overview, quarterly reports , instructions for online access, contact information

Legal

- Copies of power of attorney
- Copies of health care proxy
- Copies of health care directive

Internet

- A list of passwords. Okay, this list might violate the concepts of "security," but this notebook is not likely to leave the house. Remember, under duress, abilities diminish!

Travel (our passion)

Airline frequent flyer info
Copy of passports
Checklist for closing up our residence before travel

How to get started

Start by recognizing the value of this loving, caring tool. Get a notebook, dividers, and three-hole punch. Get a box or basket as a collection spot. Decide on a place to keep the notebook that provides easy access. It helps if it's visible in a routine work spot where mail is processed. This notebook will not likely leave the house, so don't worry about privacy or identity theft. Not having the information readily available is a bigger problem. It would cause the stress of "Where do I find this?"

Start collecting, punching, and sorting. The notebook will build over time. Make a trip to the car to find the documents in your glovebox. Search out more documents, as you think of them or need them.

The notebook can become an amazing system that keeps goals in focus and future expenditures in view, but most people don't have the mental energy at the end of a busy day to implement the system to the nth degree.

It's easy to just do what's needed with good intention for better organization later. Find a rhythm that works for you. We don't attend to this notebook daily. We put into a bin any papers that need to be filed. Once a quarter we bring out the notebook, a hole punch, and the bin, put on a light movie, and get the job done.

May this Homefront notebook be a good exercise in organization, and may your life proceed "happily ever after."

Best wishes for your good life ahead!

A Reminder To Breathe And Exercise

Healthy am I. Happy am I. Holy am I.
Whole and balanced...in mind, body and spirit.
- Jupp's suggested meditation.

Shortly after his diagnosis, my new cancer friend, Jim said he observed that he wasn't breathing. Clearly, breathing is essential to life. He probably meant he noticed that he was breathing shallowly, a symptom of the anxiety. To his credit he was aware of what was happening in his body. Our breath reveals a lot about our current state of mind. When we're uncomfortable, stressed, anxious, or fearful, we may find ourselves breathing very shallowly. When we're relaxed, we breathe slowly.

A Tutorial on Breathing: It's that important!

Our friend, Jupp Gill, a certified yoga instructor in the Greater San Francisco area, offered breath training as a valuable tool to help restore balance of body and mind. Jupp is from the Gill family who brought us the Chardi Kala philosophy. His good energy and big heart offered much to maximize our efforts. This young man of Punjabi background blends modern thinking and science with sensitivity to the ancient ways of his heritage. He encourages yoga as a life practice for men. His special efforts include yoga work with the stressed and distressed in our communities. He leads yoga programs with incarcerated young men, works with teens, reaches out to the homeless.

He expounded on the many benefits of a practice of simple, deep breathing. Conscious breathing delivers nourishing oxygen needed in every cell of our body. It aids in the removal of carbon dioxide from the bloodstream through the lungs. It helps the lymphatic system to drain. It's something you can do to help to those red blood cells who may be floundering in dysfunction! Load them up with oxygen. Don't make them work harder through shallow breathing.

Breathing slowly and deeply into the belly opens up your lungs. Open lungs reduce prospects of bacteria finding a warm, dark fold to start colonizing. Pneumonia can take hold in those little creases that occur when your lungs don't fully inflate. Pneumonia means more medications for a longer period of time. It's an additional strain to your floundering immune system. Do what you can to dodge the pneumonia bullet. If 5 minutes of deep breathing helps, what do you have to lose?

Paying attention to the quality of your breath gives insight into your sense of well-being. As Jim indicated above, shallow breathing is often a sign of anxiety. Conscious breathing can reduce stress and help muscles to relax. It can lower blood pressure as well as improve other physiological systems. Deep breathing can help alleviate pain. Anticipate pain and you tend to hold your breath. Breathe into the pain and muscles relax, oxygen flows, CO_2 is removed. It all helps.

Different breathing techniques can address different kinds of stress.

Alternate nose breathing is helpful when you feel anxious or ungrounded. There is lots of science about this practice and the effect on the balance of the nervous system. Air through one nostril stimulates. Air through the other relaxes. Measured breathing between both sides strives for balance. Hold your right thumb over your right nostril and inhale deeply through your left nostril. At the peak of your inhalation, close off your left nostril with your fourth finger, lift your right thumb, and then exhale smoothly through your right nostril. After a full exhalation, inhale through the right nostril, closing it off with your right thumb at the peak of your inhalation, lift your fourth finger and exhale smoothly through your left nostril. The science term for this is "valving". Continue with this practice for 3 to 5 minutes, alternating your breathing through each nostril. The added dimension of your coordinated hand movement helps the focus and the rhythm.

Ocean's Breath is suggested to settle your mind when you feel angry, irritated, or frustrated. This practice adds auditory feedback, additional stimulus that relaxes tension by flexing small muscles in the throat and chest. Inhale slightly deeper than normal. With your mouth closed, exhale through your nose while gently constricting your throat muscles. Try exhaling the sound "haaaaah" with your mouth open or think of it as fogging a mirror. Now make a similar sound with your mouth closed, feeling the outflow of air through your nasal passages. Once you have mastered this on the outflow, use the same method for the inflow breath, gently constricting your throat as you inhale. If you are doing this correctly, you should sound like waves on the ocean.

Gather all the tools, techniques and processes you can that will help you in this fight. And don't forget to breathe!

Okay, one more shot at promoting the importance and benefits of exercise.

Here are three articles found by a general search. We want you to know that the importance of exercise is backed by high science.

The Effects of Exercise on Bone Marrow: www.fightaging.org/archives/2011/09/the-effects-of-exercise-on-bone-marrow

"Working out influences stem cells to become bone instead of fat, improving overall health by boosting the body's capacity to make blood."

"Some of the impact of exercise is comparable to what we see with pharmaceutical intervention."

Exercise promotes bone marrow cell survival and recipient reconstitution post bone marrow transplantation, which is associated with increased survival:

http://www.exphem.org/article/S0301-472X(12)00432-8/abstract

"Exercise training increases recipient survival after BMT with increased total blood cell reconstitution."

Exercise and Bone Marrow Transplantation: http://www.bone-marrowmx.com/exercise-and-bone-marrow-transplantation

"Exercising throughout treatment and after a bone marrow transplant or stem cell transplant can increase the recovery period, boost the production of new healthy bone marrow cells, and help stimulate the immune system."

What's your exercise plan? What's your exercise commitment?

Thanks For Your Love And Support

We were very fortunate to live only four miles from Huntsman Cancer Institute, a unique, world-class cancer center. As noted on the Huntsman Cancer Institute website, "Jon Huntsman, Sr., has had cancer four times, so he's spent enough time in cancer hospitals to know what he'd do differently when he designed one from scratch. That's why Huntsman Cancer Institute is unlike any other. It looks different. It feels different."

Thanks to my Salt Lake City cousin, Bob, and his wife, Sue, who were the regulars we needed. They provided a contact with "normal" life. They brought outside social connections with good conversation about family news, community events, local politics, and suggested books. They provided normalcy. Everybody needs a Bob and Sue.

Thanks to the Gill family who brought us principles of Sikhism, a different way of thinking that gave us focus, philosophy and strength.

Thanks to our friends, the Howells. Jerry survived two major cancer traumas, and Claudia pushed through a cancer challenge of her own. They knew how and when to cluster around us and provide diversion or reward. They gathered us in when bad news loomed, mentally preparing us for what might be ahead. They celebrated with us on the ski slopes when goals were reached.

Jerry recommended the book *Love, Medicine & Miracles, Lessons Learned about Self-healing from a Surgeon's Experience with Exceptional Patients* by Bernie S. Siegel, MD. Jerry provided the following message and motivation to work through the book when our thinking was scattered: have hope and take control of your life.

Thanks to Jerry for motivating us to write this book. Their survival has honed Jerry's sense of "Paying It Forward."

Thanks to Carol and Linda for their support to keep my career alive while I was going through my treatments. I will never be able to adequately express my appreciation.

Thanks to Joel for his continuous drive to keep me positive.

Thanks to Josh for keeping Kathy's side of the business running while she provided caregiver support.

Thanks to family and friends for your frequent messages of emotional and spiritual support. The daily flow of e-mail messages gave each day meaning. You all took good care of me from near and far.

Thanks to everyone at Huntsman Cancer Institute! Amazing people take on this work.

We are all stronger together.

Resources and References

Books

From This Moment On—On Receiving the Diagnosis of Cancer by Arlene Cotter

This book is sharp and clear yet calming and nourishing. It's nicely paced with generally one idea at a time expressed in text and art. Open to any page and find a strong, soothing, or enlightening idea. It can stimulate your thinking and give you food for thought for your internal journal.

Love, Medicine & Miracles, Lessons Learned about Self-healing from a Surgeon's Experience with Exceptional Patients by Bernie S. Siegel, MD

"Unconditional love is the most powerful stimulant of the immune system. The truth is love heals. Miracles happen to exceptional patients every day—patients who have the courage to love, those who have the courage to work with their doctors to participate in and influence their own recovery."

A Conversation with My Children: A Guided Journal for Parents to Share their Story & Heart with their Adult Children by Terrika Faciane

"This guided journal will be a place to let your life speak; to leave a living legacy for your children and grandchildren. Your story matters, and no one can share it better than you.

"Use this resource as a place to let your adult children know where you came from and the love and the vision that you held (and hold) for them. May you have the freedom to impart all you have had a desire to share but wondered if it were too late or even necessary.

"Feel at liberty to reveal the wisdom and counsel you wish had been shared with you. Share the things that would help you feel lighter and make your children's life clearer if they just understood *this* or *that* reality about your journey.

"May you embrace and enjoy the journey of sharing and expressing your story, hopes, and vision with your children, and may you all experience clarity, healing (if need be) and wholeness as a result.

Memories for My Child by Peter Pauper Press

"Record details of your life, family history, values, memories, and more for your children by following the prompts in this appealing keepsake journal.

With sections for school and work, marriage and spirituality and, of course, parenthood, the guided questions here will help you create a family heirloom.

Inside back cover pocket holds keepsakes, notes.

Creamy smooth paper takes pen beautifully.

Archival, acid-free paper helps preserve precious memories."

BeTheMatch.org, *operated by the National Marrow Donor Program (NMDP)*

Be The Match offers many free programs and resources to support patients, caregivers, and family members before, during, and after transplant. Connect with Be The Match in the way that works best for you.

ONLINE: BeTheMatch.org/patient

REQUEST INFORMATION: BeTheMatch.org/request

E-MAIL: patientinfo@nmdp.org

PHONE: 1 (888) 999-6743

MASK - SPORTSTA MASK (www.johnnyrunner.com)

CPSIA information can be obtained
at www.ICGtesting.com
Printed in the USA
FFHW022217140119
50172925-55103FF